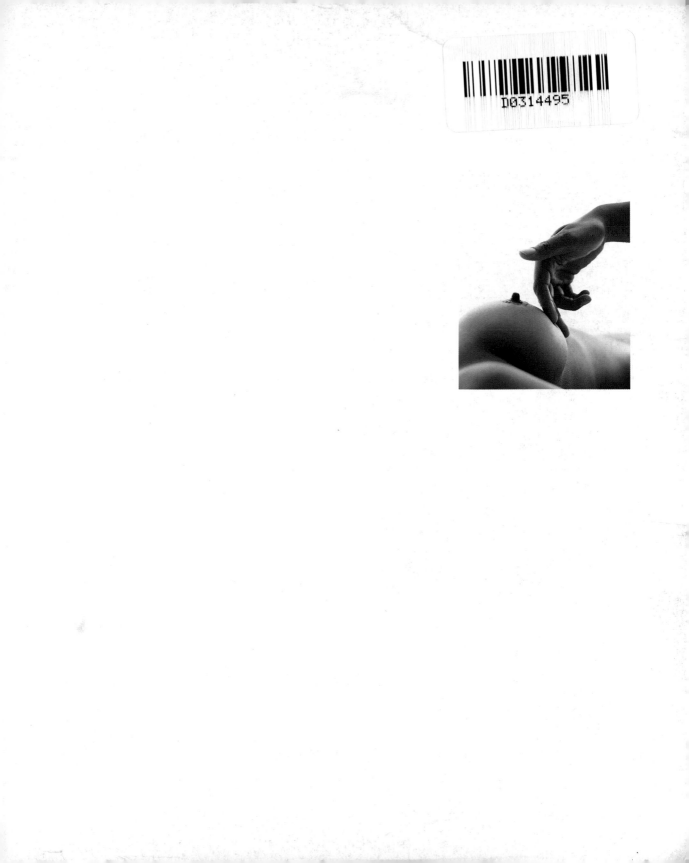

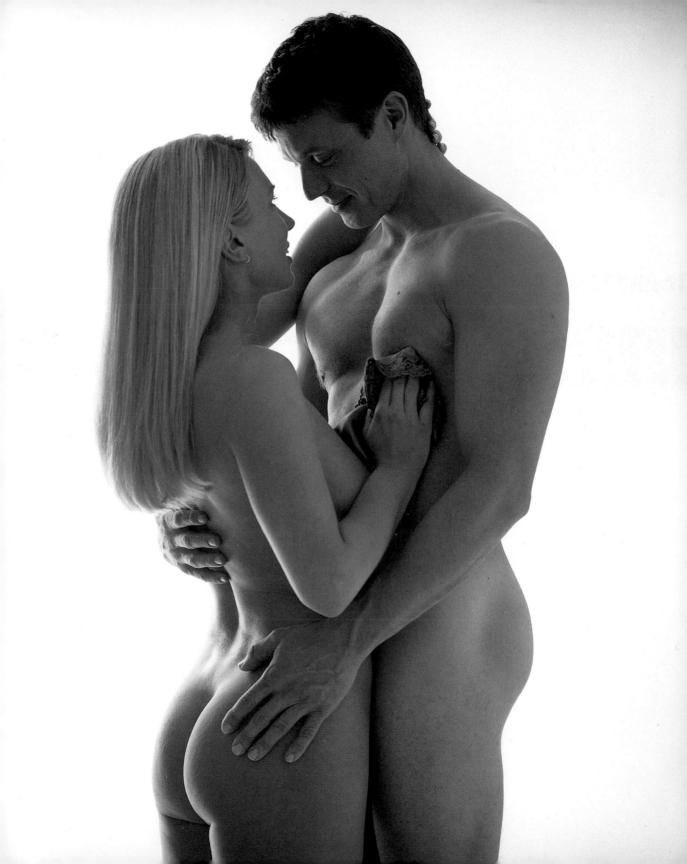

Dr Andrew Stanway

massagesecrets
for lovers

the ultimate guide to intimate arousal

Quadrille

First published in 2002 by Quadrille Publishing Limited
Alhambra House
27–31 Charing Cross Road
London WC2H OLS

Editorial Director: **Jane O'Shea**
Creative Director: **Mary Evans**
Art Editor: **Rachel Gibson**
Project Editor: **Mary Davies**
Production: **Nancy Roberts**

Photography: **Jules Selmes**
Illustrations: **John Gearey**

Cataloguing-in-Publication Data: a catalogue record for this book is
available from the British Library.

ISBN 1 903845 87 4

Printed and bound in Spain

contents

foreword

Many couples make some sort of massage a part of their loving life together. Most sensual massage, though, however delightful, could be done to your child, or even your grandmother!

Erotic massage is an entirely different matter. It's a sexy event between lovers, whose purpose is a combination of erotic pleasure, sexual arousal, orgasm, spiritual connection, and possibly intercourse. The aim, in other words, is to use whatever you find effective and pleasurable to delight your partner, to turn them on, and almost certainly to arouse yourself. It is frankly and obviously a form of lovemaking – but one that works on a rather higher plane than most day-to-day sexual encounters.

what? better than sex?

Over the years I've spent thousands of hours listening to couples being honest about their sex lives and relationships. Most of them say the sex is great on about two occasions out of ten, a failure or disappointing on another two, and OK the rest of the time. *Massage Secrets for Lovers* is a way of upping the odds to where perhaps half the time your lovemaking is really great. And that would be a vast improvement for most of us.

As a culture, we've become too hooked on intercourse as the main way of 'making' love. The truth, I'm afraid, is that for much of the time the average, even quite 'together' couple doesn't so much make love as 'have sex'. This, to put it crudely, often means using the genitals of their partner to masturbate their own. Small wonder things don't go too well or that many people get bored, look elsewhere and start to have problems with sex or their relationship.

Erotic massage works on an entirely different plane. The 'making of love', as I call it, becomes a whole-body/mind/spirit event that soars above the average sex session. But this doesn't just happen without some knowledge, insight and effort.

At this point many people will throw up their hands and complain that lovemaking should be spontaneous, fun and uncontrived … and that they really don't want or need yet another set of tasks to cope with in their already over-stressed, over-stretched and goal-centred lives.

I understand this point of view entirely. But one person's stressful 'goal' is another's delicious journey of discovery. It's a matter of perception. And I believe that this book can help you see the learning process as something to enjoy. After all, you wouldn't have read even this far if you weren't interested in advancing your love live. This is bound to take at least some time and effort.

The beauty of this journey, though, is that results are apparent right from the start. Unlike learning to play the violin, where you can spend years getting halfway good and in the meantime are just a nuisance to others, erotic massage opens doors very quickly to a better life together, both in and out of the bedroom.

what? no sex?

The clinical experience of professionals such as myself is that intercourse rates are falling throughout the Western world, and have been doing so for two decades. People are busier, women are more tired, couples have other priorities, sex is seen as less fulfilling than other things they could be doing, many of us want instant pleasure, preferably without much personal effort – the reasons are numerous.

Erotic massage comes to the rescue in a world like this. Whether you're off sex for some medical reason, are pregnant and don't fancy it, are worried that you or your partner has a sexually transmitted infection, if you have any sort of sexual dysfunction, or are bored in bed, erotic massage can provide an exciting and rewarding alternative.

But it is much more than this. Erotic massage can build a whole new dimension of spiritual and emotional connection that many couples never, or rarely, experience through intercourse. We are raised in a culture that talks of sex as if it were a consumer commodity – something that can be obtained, like a washing machine. But true sexual delight and rewarding relationships are the result of a long-term commitment to working together to create something of value that can't be 'bought'.

It depends what you're after. If you simply want to scratch a sexual itch, this book will probably annoy you. But if you're looking to enhance your loving and sexual life with your special person and if you want to empower yourself outside the bedroom by releasing parts of your inner self you never knew were there, then you'll love it.

And this is important. In a loving relationship, if I seek to pleasure and honour my partner, I myself grow. Nothing in *Massage Secrets for Lovers* involves a path of selfless devotion to your lover at the expense of yourself. It really is a give-to-get book and one where both of you will benefit right from the start.

Dr Andrew Stanway
London, 2002

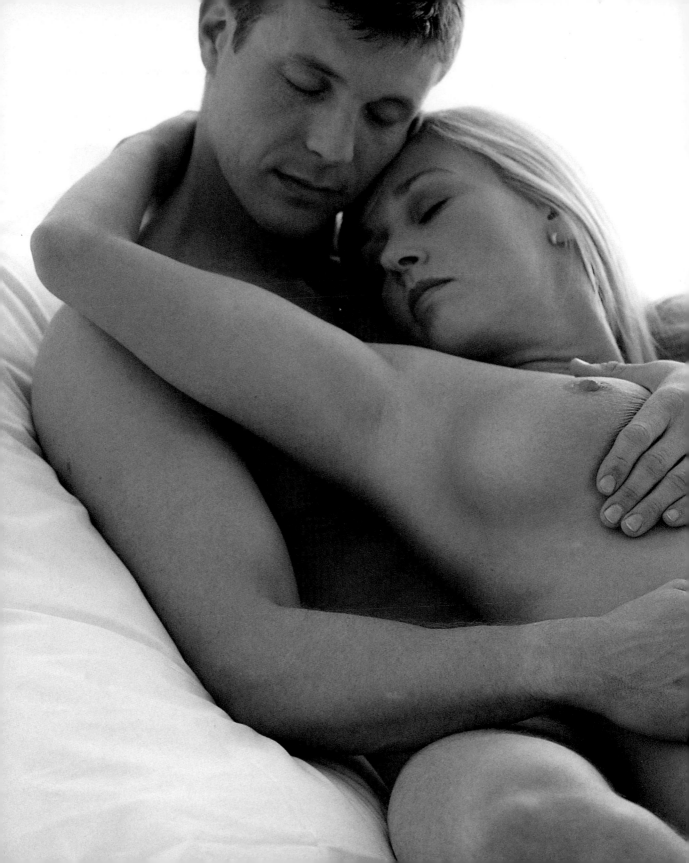

It's possible to be entirely spontaneous in how you prepare for and do an erotic massage, but my experience with couples shows me it's helpful to have some common ground between you before you start. Part One will, I hope, provide areas for discussion — even dispute — and help you both to get your heads round the subject before you involve your bodies.

part one getting ready

Finding common ground involves understanding a little of what you're aiming for at the mind and spirit level, learning a whole new way of communicating, and having a basic knowledge of the essential elements of sexual arousal. Recent research into female anatomy, for example, has changed the way we think about women's sexuality and arousal and no modern couple should be ignorant of these facts.

Of course, as throughout the book, you'll come with your own ideas and experiences, all of which are valuable to you. What I try to do here is to challenge some of these long-held 'truths' and assumptions with the intention of sharing the insights you'll need to move forward. And this, I hope, will take your familiar erotic games to a higher plane.

ancient wisdoms – new lessons

It's probably fair to say that the Western world has only really woken up to the spiritual nature of sexuality over the last few decades. For many hundreds of years somewhat mechanistic medical and scientific models largely drove the study and understanding of sex, leaving most people who ever gave the matter any thought unsatisfied because they knew deep down that there was so much more to sex than the practical know-how of what I call the 'genital plumbing'.

The East, in contrast, has always known that sexuality works on many levels … of which the mechanical is probably the least important. Taoist philosophy from ancient China and Tantric religious beliefs from India, dating back thousands of years, encouraged people to see themselves as a complex package of sexual sensuality, mysticism and spirituality. The Karma Sutra, for example, is not at all the sexual aerobics handbook it is portrayed as by the West, but a study of sexual manners, a cultured man's guide for life, in which sexual positions play only a very small part.

true intimacy

Tantra and Taoism, being largely mystical in their focus, claim that during a sensual or erotic massage it's much less important what your hands are doing than how your heart and spirit are engaged. This means that unlike a massage for a sore back or aching shoulders – either of which could be carried out with some success by anyone with the right skills – erotic massage between lovers calls for a level of communication that goes well beyond any physical manoeuvres either, or both, may perform.

From this perspective, erotic massage is an almost 'holy' experience, connecting us with parts of our lover's soul (or being) that rarely come into play during 'normal' sex. Our 'connected' bodies become a shrine to our love. Flesh becomes spirit, and the Western perception of the duality of body and soul is cancelled in a mystical dimension we inhabit together. It's an approach that frees us up to be truly intimate. And this is what erotic massage is all about.

Taoism also makes much of uninhibited, natural spontaneity. In the West we've become so hidebound by conventions, inhibitions, anxieties and guilt that it's often hard to get past this armour plating to the real person beneath. The secret here is to learn to trust your deepest intuitions and to act on the feelings of the moment rather than on 'givens' from the past. Taoist philosophers have it right when they tell us not to strive too hard – rather to 'go with the flow' and to relish the naturalness that's within us all. Unfortunately, many of us find this hard to do.

But some of the most impressive lessons to be learned from oriental philosophies are simple enough – we've just lost sight of them in our crazy modern lives. We are all capable of so much more than we think, and most of us have become lazy and take one another for granted.

How often do you consciously engage even some of your senses when making love? When did you last really smell your lover's skin? When did you listen to their breathing? When did you concentrate on the different textures of the various parts of their body? Modern life dulls our senses and we are the poorer for it. Yet in the privacy of our one-to-one love life we can re-awaken these delights and unlock a wonderful world of pleasure, relaxation and fun.

yin and yang

Few of us can honestly say we know what attracts us to our partner. Of course, there are the obvious things but these are never explanation enough. Deep down there are other intangible, 'unknowable' things. Perhaps pheromones play a part. Perhaps we can read one another's minds in ways as yet not understood by science. Perhaps, as therapists such as myself assert, we unconsciously choose someone who'll enable us to work out our deepest pains and complete our unfinished psychological 'business'.

Whatever's going on, and whether our lover is the same or the opposite gender, any relationship is shaped by a coming together of two deeply rooted, complementary principles. The 'making of love' involves a relationship between these two unconscious yet nonetheless vitally important parts of each of us.

All nature reflects this coupling – dark and light, hot and cold, dry and wet, positive and negative, male and female – a concept the ancient Chinese called yin and yang. This union of opposites is represented in the yin yang symbol (see left): the black yin (feminine) form interlocks with the white yang (masculine) form, each of them containing a dot of the other's colour.

Psychologist Carl Jung made much of this concept in his writings. Within each of us, he said, is the essence of the opposite sex. No biological system is entirely yin or yang, just as no person is entirely masculine or feminine … however genetically male or female they may be.

Understanding and accepting this underlying truth is even more vital today. In spite of the huge success of books about men being from Mars and women from Venus, loving partners know deep in their hearts that they embody not just the characteristics of their own sex but some of those of the opposite sex too. Self-aware people don't blame the opposite sex for the innermost parts that they'd rather disown. Nor do they strenuously, if unconsciously, attribute them to others. Being at one with the conflicting elements in our personalities is a sign of true maturity … and a great start for becoming spiritual lovers.

the power of chi

Eastern beliefs and philosophies place great value on understanding body energies, what the Chinese call chi (pronounced chee). Chi or vitality, it is thought, maintains, protects and transforms the body through every stage of life. Carried by invisible channels that link together every part of the body, both internally and externally, it embodies, though unseen, a physical reality essential for the harmonious balance of yin and yang. In addition to the channels that run throughout the body, there are seven areas (right) where energy is especially concentrated. These are called the chakras.

Imagine a domestic hosepipe. Water should flow smoothly through it from one end to the other. If it is kinked or blocked, the water backs up and the garden doesn't get watered. So it is with energy and the chakras. Such kinks or 'blockages' can result from adverse past experiences, from physical, mental or spiritual ill health, from sexual dysfunctions, and much more.

Most Eastern healing systems involve unblocking these kinks so that energy can flow smoothly though the chakras – the junctions in the pipe – once again. Aromatherapy, crystal healing, acupuncture, meditation, visualization, martial arts, yoga, t'ai chi, and certain body therapies are all used to re-balance the chakras.

gaining more chi through lovemaking

The second (sacral) chakra is seen as the main focus of sexual energy. It is situated at the lowest part of the spine, near the 'tail' (coccyx), and governs the sex organs and bladder, and emotional issues surrounding these organs. Problems with this chakra lead, among other things, to impotence, loss of libido, infertility and sexual addiction. Massaging a lover over the sacral chakra is believed to help rebalance sexual energies.

Taoists regard the pelvic floor and perineum (see page 108) as the lower diaphragm of the body (the upper one shuts off the lungs from the abdominal cavity). They believe that controlling the muscles of this area of the body – and that includes those of the pelvic floor, those around the urethra, vagina and anus, and the many other involuntary muscles – creates a muscle or pump for sexual energy.

When we have an orgasm, most Eastern thinking goes, the energy produced pours out into the universe and is lost to us personally. Taoist and Tantric teaching, however, aims to recycle the energy generated in our genitals back into our own body and that of our lover. This might sound simple but is, in reality, highly complicated.

Whole books have been written on the subject, and in my experience it's very difficult to achieve unless you put in a huge amount of time and effort, or, ideally, have a good teacher. Clearly it is well beyond the scope of this book.

Although many of these beliefs may sound strange, even weird, to most westerners, I believe that sexual energies do indeed circulate round the body and that over the years we'll discover ways of proving it. On pages 60–1 I describe a breast massage that a woman can use to release her own healing sexual energies. And, whatever the explanation, it is my professional experience that people whose sexual 'muscle' is poorly developed or weak do, in fact, have problems with their sexual life and don't get the sexual energy they could from their orgasms. (For details of Kegel exercises, an extremely effective way of strengthening the muscles of the pelvic floor, see page 72.)

harmonizing and connecting

We in the West can learn much from the Eastern tradition that erotic and sensual massage creates a sense of oneness with our lover. But how does this translate into immediate terms we can understand? What sort of qualities and experience do we need to achieve that oneness?

● **Love** I believe it's difficult, even impossible, to massage one another erotically without love. Not just what I call the 'love-ing' feelings that can produce great physical sensations but a deeper love that creates a meeting of souls.

● **An open body** This is vital. Many of us are so armour-plated in response to past adverse experiences that we aren't truly able to accept even the most lovingly offered touch. In my work with couples I've found that this armour can be softened, and even dissolved, by erotic massage lovingly performed.

● **An open heart** By this I mean total trust. Trust that you won't be used or abused. Trust that your uniqueness will be honoured. Trust that you'll be listened to. Trust that your lover will do the very best for you – and, if in doubt, will put your needs first.

● **A spiritual connection** Couples who think and feel along with one another, who share a sixth sense, who share dreams, who know what the other is about to say, who communicate in ways that go beyond speech are working together at a spiritual level that makes man–woman relationships magical and unbeatable. Erotic massage is a great playground for these skills.

● **Self-knowledge** Without this, we are unlikely to get the best out of a session – or indeed to give it our best. The quest for self-knowledge is a life-long one but Part Two can help you start if this is a new journey for you.

● **Practical knowledge and skills** Little will happen without these. Learning first on your own and then with your lover is part of the journey you're embarked upon together.

A good way to get in the mood for a spiritual exchange is to try to connect with one another's energy fields very deeply. The simple sequences opposite can be done before a massage session and will help harmonize your energies in preparation for true intimacy. Experiment to see which suits you best. (You don't need massage oil for either.) Some couples say they also like to use these techniques after intercourse.

total body contact

1 Ask your lover to lie on his back, with his legs apart. He must be comfortable so don't choose a hard surface.

2 Lie on top of him with your legs together so that your pelvis is over his.

3 Hold one another firmly and kiss deeply. Then relax and breathe deeply.

4 Ignore his erection. Simply focus on maximum skin-to-skin contact and your loving feelings for one another.

● **Variation** Ask your man to lie face down. Lie with your front on his back, holding him firmly as you both focus on loving contact.

channelling energies

1 Ask your lover to lie face down in a comfortable position. Rub your palms briskly together several times to build up warmth and energy in them. Focusing your energy into your hands will help you 'break through' the aura or energy field that surrounds your partner's body more gently. Enriching your hand-energy also makes for a more rewarding massage.

2 Place the palm of one hand on the base of your lover's spine and the palm of the other at the top of the spine, near the base of their neck.

3 Close your eyes, relax, breathe deeply and tune in to your partner.

4 Match your breathing and try to pick up what your partner is feeling.

5 Think loving thoughts about your partner and 'send' them through your hands.

6 Imagine sending a stream of energy in a circle from your left hand to your right, via your heart, your arms and your partner's spine. Ask your lover to imagine the energy flow with you. Some actually describe the flow so that their partner can visualize it better. This takes practice so be patient.

changing attitudes

There are several sections later in Part One that suggest practical ways in which you can both get ready for erotic massage. Here, I'll look briefly at ways you may need to change your attitudes to the making of love.

isn't it too late to change?

To get the best out of erotic massage you must believe you can have more intense, longer-lasting orgasms that produce more pleasure. Strangely, this can be difficult. For most of us, perception and expectation are limited by our current situation, especially if those ways of thinking have been entrenched in our psyche over many years. This often prejudices us against new or 'higher' pleasures. Others of us have come to believe that our lovers limit our pleasure. If only they were 'better at it', we'd have more fun. This may, of course, be true but it is far more likely that we unwittingly limit ourselves. It can be helpful to discuss these issues calmly some time … though not during a massage session! To do this successfully, you'll need lots of empathic listening skills (see pages 20–1).

what's in it for me?

It's human nature to be somewhat selfish. Many couples I teach ask the question, 'What's in it for me?' My answer is, 'a satisfied partner'. A lover who is happy and satisfied is more likely to return sensual or sexual favours.

Some people are more altruistic than others but few of us can accept one-way traffic for long, and problems arise in many relationships when one partner finds themselves consistently doing more giving. This can lead to bad feelings or even bitterness, as the other seems to do most of the taking. Of course, that partner may not be greedier or more selfish. The aggrieved one who is apparently short-changed often has all kinds of unconscious inhibitions on receiving pleasure, or has too limited a view of pleasure. And that may not be the other's fault.

Pain and pleasure are thought of as opposites but they are really much the same in that they both flood our senses, demanding our full attention. For a person for whom 'pain', however defined, feels wrong, guilt-inducing, shameful, unloving or whatever, 'pleasure' or massive orgasm can be elusive, no matter how loving or able their partner is. This can be very frustrating for both parties.

when do I have my turn?

It's your 'turn' whenever you do something wonderful to your lover. You don't have to be 'done to' to be having a turn. I look at this in more detail later (see giving and receiving, pages 18–19). It might sound rather 'noble', or even unlikely, but the highest rewards and delights come from doing for your partner the best you can. And that's the secret of great erotic massage. It really is Give to Get.

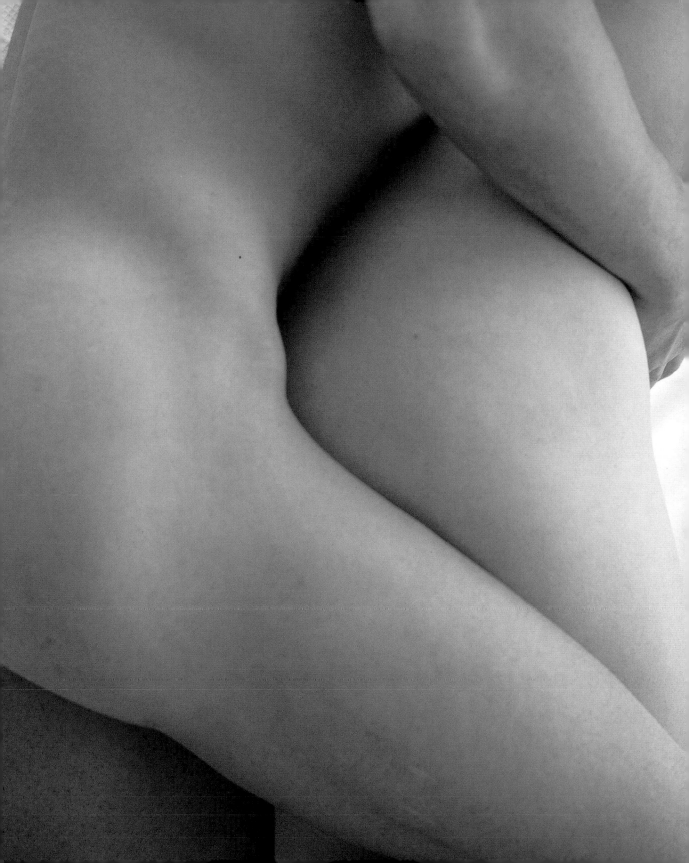

giving and receiving

There are few relationships in life in which both parties find it equally easy to give and receive. Some of us are conditioned to be 'givers' and others 'takers'. Such behaviour patterns obviously find a place in the bedroom – and you'll probably find yourself doing more giving and receiving than ever before as you practise your erotic massage skills. If you really want to get the best out of giving and receiving, it helps to have a little insight into what's going on.

rescuers and victims

Many people who are apparently selfless givers are, in fact, 'rescuers'. By this I mean they unconsciously try to rescue their lovers from their pains and difficulties in life. This might, at first, sound great. But it usually isn't because rescuers rescue others to avoid rescuing themselves from their own unhappy stuff and the receiver often ends up feeling like a victim. That's neither sexy nor comfortable. And it's no basis for a truly intimate relationship. If you feel this might apply to your relationship, talk it through with your partner sometime when you're feeling positive towards one another. If necessary, seek professional help.

giving is receiving

Many people have difficulty recognizing that in a loving, intimate relationship giving and receiving happen simultaneously. The receiver gives total trust to the giver who, in turn, becomes completely open and sensitive to needs of the receiver. By giving, we receive – and vice versa. In a sense, everything we do for our lover, we do for ourselves. It's a delicious paradox. As we pleasure and enrich them, we ourselves grow. Erotic massage that's working well is about sharing both energy flows and communication.

Many people in today's busy, ego-centred world find it harder to receive than to give. Most of us are so used to 'doing' all the time that erotic massage can be seen as yet another chore – however pleasurable – that we have to 'do'.

When receiving, try to be completely receptive. Shut off the outside world, apart from your lover, and focus on the moment and all your bodily sensations. Your only job is to let your lover know what's nice and what isn't. Your only responsibility is to be a loving guide. And it is a responsibility because without your guidance your partner won't know what's going on, especially in the early days. And this isn't fair. No one can read your mind. You have to say, or communicate in non-verbal ways, exactly what you like or want. I've lost count of the number of couples I've seen who expect one another to be psychic, and then get annoyed when their partner is not (see learning to be a good guide, page 23).

exchanging roles

In many relationships it's the woman who takes control of 'emotional matters' and the man of more physical concerns. Erotic massage is the ideal context in which to adjust this balance. Because it offers high returns in the pleasure stakes many men find themselves able to be more truly intimate during a massage session than they usually would be. But this can happen only if women give them space to do so. It's important, therefore, that a woman doesn't unwittingly shut her man out of emotional expression and release just because in everyday life she sees this as her territory. My clinical experience is that most men, given 'permission' by their partner, feel free to engage in issues that demand emotional intelligence. In fact, I've used erotic massage as a key to achieving this in many couples.

different modes — different rewards

One of the most fascinating things about being a relationship therapist is observing how couples communicate — and relaying this back to them. One or other partner is usually more verbal, uses and observes body language more, emotes more, or thinks more, and so on. True communication occurs when both parties are operating in the same mode. And again this is where erotic massage can be so helpful. Because the sexual thrill and the desire to please one another are so great, it's a good stage on which to learn to read one another's communication modes … and then tailor-make your own to create the most effective exchange. In a sense this is what this whole book is about.

communication skills

By now it will be clear that the physical intimacy lovers experience during erotic massage is only part of the story. Most people enjoy this kind of massage because it takes them beyond pleasant bodily sensations.

When we massage one another erotically, we're open to a level of communication that we rarely experience, even when having sex. That's why it's helpful to know how to be truly intimate with one another, especially when, for many lovers, novel bodily pleasures and experiences seem to unlock all kinds of hidden emotions. These will need to be carefully and lovingly dealt with if you want to build your relationship through erotic massage.

I have found that couples can only do this really effectively if they know how to listen empathically to one another. But leaving such learning until you're in the thick of erotic massage thrills isn't wise. And be aware – empathic listening could take weeks, even months, to perfect. Once you know you can truly listen to your lover, who'll feel loved and understood as a result, it's time to consider two other communication skills you need to get the best out of your erotic massage sessions: taking care of your partner, and being a good guide.

empathic listening

Empathy is different from sympathy. If I'm being empathic with you, I put myself in your shoes and try to imagine what it's like being you. I can, with practice, actually enter into your being and feel things alongside you. This enables me to deal with your emotions not in the way I deal with mine own, but from inside you. When I'm being sympathetic with you, my focus is on how I feel and that does you no good. The distinction is important because when I am listening to you empathically you feel truly understood. So how can you learn this technique? By recognizing and practising the three elements involved.

● **Put your own ego to one side.** Try to block out thoughts of yourself and your feelings about the topic under discussion and listen solely to your partner. This can be very difficult in an ego-centred culture such as ours but can be achieved with practice and motivation.

● **Identify your lover's main emotion.** The skill here is to observe the body language closely, to listen with your 'third ear' to what's actually being said rather than what the voice is saying, and to tune in to everything that you know about

your partner. Most of us feel confused when we experience several emotions at once. A partner who can help us identify our main emotion does us a great service.

● **Reflect that emotion back to your partner.** There are no prizes for simply being able to name what your partner is feeling. Your value lies in offering back what you think this is. If you say, 'You're obviously feeling angry' and they're not, then you've lost an opportunity. Try making an offering like: 'It seems to me you're feeling angry'. If they are, fine.

They'll feel understood, more able to recognize their own emotions and thus to have some control over them. If they're not, they can gently correct you by saying, 'It's not exactly anger. It's more like lonely' … or whatever else they are feeling. This helps them define what they are feeling and helps you understand how they look, sound, feel and so on when they are feeling lonely. And you'll both have learned something really valuable from this encounter – which may have lasted less than a minute. It is amazing how much can be achieved in so short a time if you are truly open to listening with your 'third ear'.

If all this sounds contrived, that's because it is! But it needs to be until empathic listening becomes a habit for you both. After only a few weeks of practising this type of soul-to-soul listening, you'll find your erotic massage sessions take on a very different 'colour'. And what you learn here will affect the whole of your life together.

taking care of your partner

We all need to feel totally safe if we are to relax into pleasure during erotic massage. This means the giver must take responsibility for the whole environment and for practical things, such as any equipment they'll need, as well as phones going, doorbells ringing or children interrupting (see pages 38–41). And the receiver must know that the giver will be constantly caring and protective. There are several ways in which a giver can build and maintain that trust.

● **Agree the limits before you start.** Once you become skilled erotic lovers, you'll know these in advance, of course. But never spring surprises, however experienced you both are.

● **Keep your partner informed.** At first, explain exactly what you're going to do before each step. Once you are skilled and your partner knows what to expect, you can relax this rule. Early on, though, it makes for security, especially for those who are fearful. You may find it hard to believe that someone could be afraid of too much pleasure but some people certainly are.

● **Ask only questions that require Yes or No answers.** Avoid exam-type, multiple-choice questions that require lots of thought. Good questions are: 'Would you like this faster?' 'Is this pressure about right?' Don't ask questions such as, 'Is this nice?' The reply could offend you. Or your partner may think it might, and so lie. You can experiment in daily life with this sort of communication.

● **Don't take things for granted.** Just because something goes well once, it doesn't mean it always will. Many women, for example, find that what they enjoy varies from time to time according to where they are in their menstrual cycle; how they are feeling about themselves, their lover, or life in general; and certainly over the course of a lifetime. This means that sensitive 'listening' to your lover will be an ongoing necessity. It is a real relationship builder.

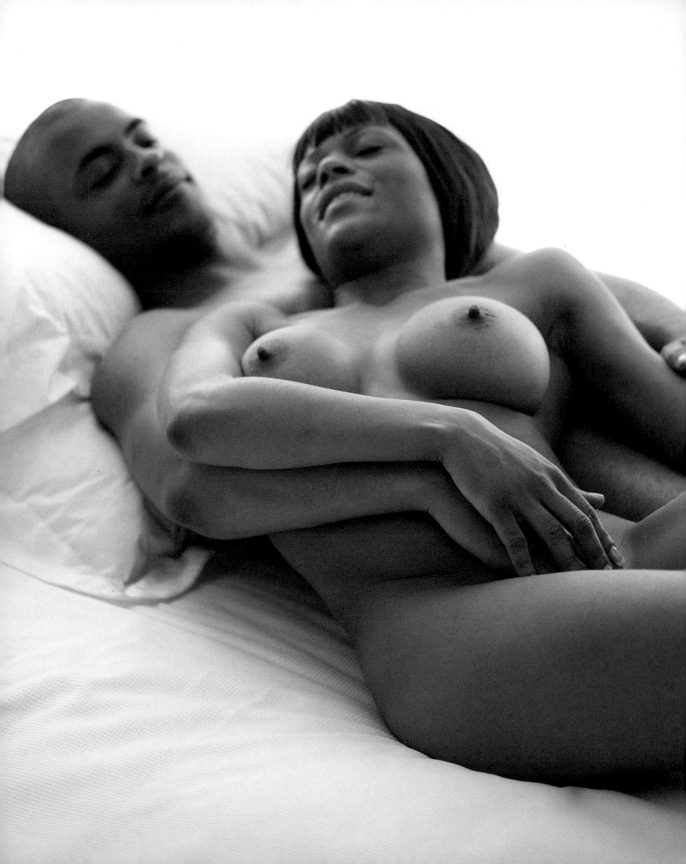

learning to be a good guide

Being a good receiver is a skill that needs a little practice if things are to go well. I find it means being a good guide. Few people like to be 'told' what to do when in bed with a lover, but most are happy to be guided.

● **Be explicit.** Many couples complain that they just don't know what it is their partner actually wants. This means both of you must take responsibility for what you do want. Ask for things directly: 'Please do that to my foot again' or 'Your fingertips feel great doing that'.

● **Give one instruction at a time.** First, this will help you decide exactly what's nicest, and, second, it'll avoid confusion.

● **Miss no opportunity to show your approval.** The more your partner has your approval the more they will try to please you and the more pleasure you'll get. This is a learned skill. It might involve actually saying something encouraging or just giving a lovely sigh or body movement that shows you're really getting what you want.

● **Try not to be critical.** Encourage the good rather than criticize the 'bad'. If your partner is going too fast or too hard, ask for what you want. Too many couples find themselves getting poor results because one or both are so negative about even the tiniest thing that goes wrong. Be gentle with one another.

● **Talk about things afterwards.** This makes the experience 'real' for you both, summarizes what you've felt, helps decide what you'd like to repeat and what you wouldn't, and cements the uniqueness of the event as part of your loving life together. Many people tell me it's hard to talk about even very enjoyable sensations afterwards but clinical experience shows me it is really helpful. And it's a practice that can make it easier for you to communicate about all sorts of things in life.

setting up a scoring system

Because sexual arousal and pleasure are so compelling, and because we're disinclined to be analytical about sex on the principle 'If it ain't broke, don't fix it', most of us find it difficult to assess how aroused we are at any time. And that makes it hard to judge if something our lover or we are doing is having any effect.

I find it's helpful to create a scale of, say, 1 to 5 so that you can, at any time in a loving session, rate your state of arousal fairly accurately. Over the months you'll find the range of the scale will increase as you become more orgasmic and arousable but within that scale you'll still be able to place yourself from 1 to 5.

It's a trick that has real practical value for you, both as a receiver and a giver, because you can tell your partner at any time where you are or check where they are. Remember, though, that their 3 will not be your 3! Really in-tune, long-term lovers learn to score each other accurately at any time too, and this gives the receiver the confidence of being perfectly understood.

breathing to inspire

Although it's obvious that we need to breathe to sustain life, there's far more to breathing than the simple exchange of oxygen and carbon dioxide. Over my years as a body psychotherapist I have become more and more interested in the subject.

In English, the very word 'inspiration' has two highly significant meanings – to breathe in, or to be in a state of special creative activity – while the word 'expire' can mean to breathe out, or to die. And our word 'spirit' is related to the Latin verb meaning to breathe. With this background it's hardly surprising the subject is so inspiring!

Whenever I ask people where in their body they think their spirit, soul or being might reside, with very few exceptions they point to their chest. Clearly, breathing is somehow linked to the notion of connecting with, and enhancing, the spirit or being – the process that I call 'in-spirit-ation'. Indeed, some Buddhists spend many hours each day for years simply focusing on their breath as it goes in and out because they find this gives them profound insights into the nature of life, as well as being pleasurable in itself.

Chi, the Chinese name for body energy (see pages 12–13), derives from the word for breath (or air), and ancient Chinese philosophers saw breathing as the way each of us communicates with the universal energy. Now, in the twenty-first century, we know that oxygen produced by trees half a planet away finds its way into our lungs, fuels our whole metabolism and in a very real sense becomes part of us. This means that the emphasis on interconnection and interdependence isn't mumbo-jumbo, but highly practical stuff that rings perhaps even more true today than it did three thousand years ago to peoples who had a fraction of our knowledge of biochemistry and global ecology.

breathing and sex

Taoist and Tantric teaching hold that the act of love is essentially one of respiration. You breathe – both literally and metaphorically – your sexual energy into your lover's body and soul and they do the same for you. This is a skill that it takes many years to perfect but the idea itself expresses an important truth. To make the deepest connection in lovemaking, we must each surrender our sexual soul. It's a type of devotion, nourishing your lover in a way no one else can.

Try this experiment when making love one day. You're both feeling highly aroused and breathing in rhythm with one another as penis penetrates vagina. Imagine the energy as it flows back and forth from penis to vagina, from clitoris to clitoris. Think your partner's sexual energy up from your pelvis and into your head. You'll find this is greatly helped by contracting your pelvic muscles, anus and buttocks. Now in all your actions let this energy flow back to your lover as you create a loving circuit.

Many men say they can sense at once when their partner is withholding this energy. And in my clinical experience withholding on either side seems to be at the heart of many poor-quality sexual experiences. Indeed, many couples never get to experience sexual bliss, so tight are they and so unable to yield up their sexual souls.

breathing as release

The phrase 'tight-assed' has real meaning for any professional who practises body therapy. Anxiety, tension, anger, frustration and many other negative emotions show as tense pelvic muscles. The jaw muscles also seem to tighten in those who have problems with sexual arousal and letting go. Massaging the pelvic muscles directly (see pages 108–11 and 130–1) relaxes them while easing tension elsewhere in the body. But very deep breathing – filling your lungs right to the top and then breathing out fully and slowly – has a very positive effect on the pelvic diaphragm too. You can check this on yourself (or on your lover), especially when obviously tense. Just insert a finger or two into the vagina or anus and feel the tension – it may be difficult to get a finger in at all. Now breathe deeply, filling the lungs to the very top and then emptying them completely, before breathing in again. Within as few as ten breaths, you'll feel the effect as the pelvic-floor muscles begin to relax on your fingers.

Many of my patients have found deep breathing helpful in improving orgasm quality, and some women have been able to experience orgasm for the first time. I recommend a very simple breathing exercise for anyone who finds it difficult to let go. It's a version of the 'test' above. Relax your jaw and breathe deeply and slowly as you stimulate yourself to arousal. As you become more aroused, your breathing becomes quicker and shallower. Concentrate on keeping it slow and deep. You can also use breathing to delay orgasm. Focus on breathing and you'll find you can take the edge off your arousal for just a moment. With practice, it's possible to use breath awareness to create a rise and fall in your arousal level until you are ready to come.

the power of touch

The vast majority of human interactions involve little or no bodily contact, but when they do we try to control things so that we feel comfortable. All our social interactions are based on an unspoken set of 'touch-scripts'. For example, if your father-in-law were to caress your thigh, it would probably feel inappropriate and embarrassing at best – and utterly unacceptable at worst. Even someone standing too close in a crowded train can feel 'wrong'.

Of course, when we meet someone we fancy, we progress through a series of touching stages designed to test and overturn our everyday scripts. At first we touch hands – shaking hands with almost anyone of either sex isn't considered in any way threatening or inappropriate; later we embrace, and then start to kiss and caress non-genital parts of their body, and finally graduate to genital caresses and even intercourse. 'Arriving' at intercourse doesn't mean we abandon all other forms of touching. If that were the case, this book would be redundant! In fact, the loving couple continue their voyage of discovery year in, year out.

But almost all our 'touch-scripts' originate deep in our unconscious memories of baby- and early child-hood. Years of experience in bodywork psychotherapy have shown me just how rooted we are in such matters and how this governs our dealings with lovers. One person's erotic zone is another's hell zone – and so on. It's fair to say that if you or your partner has very powerful feelings about any particular part of the body and its sensations, the reason will probably lie way back in your earliest days.

Over my years as a hands-on therapist I have seen the most remarkable responses to touch. At first it amazed me just how huge the reaction could be to even the tiniest touch or hold. In fact it was these sorts of responses that led me deeper into the whole subject of body psychotherapy.

Most doctors and mental health-care professionals who don't touch people in their work find it hard to believe just how many valuable lessons can be learned from people's unconscious responses to touch. Of course, it's vital to be aware of exactly what's going on and to be open to even the tiniest changes. This can be tricky at first, especially if your lover seems distressed when you touch them. Take time out, stop what you're doing and try to discover what's happening. It's highly likely that your partner won't be able to say because many of the emotions will be pre-verbal – dating back to infantile experiences. Just hold them and channel love into them as they cry, shake, sob, laugh or scream. Being there for them could be the very best 'therapy'. If things are really difficult, don't hesitate to see a professional.

the erogenous zones

The mind is, in my view, the largest erogenous zone. Whether it's at a conscious or unconscious level, our thoughts, our fantasies and our waking or sleeping dreams all inform the mind. And it's the mind – that unique combination of experience and brain function – that causes us to appreciate the sexiness of a lover. By the time we begin to explore our partner's body we are already aroused. This process is, of course, closely linked to powerful, primitive chemical attractants, some of which are now being researched in detail. Yes, there really is a chemistry behind physical attraction. But what exactly it is will probably remain a mystery for many years to come.

In general, women are more responsive to touch than are men because their pleasure zones can include almost any area of their body. This is probably because the reproductive consequences of intercourse are so great for women – the immediate rewards of sexual contact have to be high or they'd never get involved!

Everyone, everywhere, finds the mouth, genitals and anal areas sexually arousing when caressed. Men's most erogenous zones are confined to their lips, nipples and the area covered by their underpants. But almost any area of the body can experience highly erotic sensations if stimulated in the right way by the right person. You'll discover that ears, breasts (especially nipples), inner arms and legs, and the nape of the neck are all sensitive to delicate touch. Caresses here heighten sensual pleasure and can even lead to orgasm. During soul-to-soul intercourse the whole body can become one huge erogenous zone, of course, making a nonsense of the concept of discrete zones.

inward and outward orgasms

Human orgasm is an almost spiritual concept. Ask any hundred people at random what they experience as they climax and you'll get a hundred different answers.

There are mini-orgasms and hugely powerful ones, 'mystical' or explosive ones, multiple or single ones, ejaculatory or dry ones (in both sexes), orgasms that last for a few seconds and others that go on for hours, orgasms focused on the clitoris or the genitals in general and those that seem to involve the whole body. There are those that don't involve the genitals at all and there are even out-of-body orgasms.

When I was working with another therapist in the 1980s we listed between us well over a hundred ways women could experience orgasm. Some did so from non-genital sources. For example, some could climax on hearing a lover's voice on the telephone, some on being afraid, others on having their feet massaged, and even one on combing her hair! A very few could just think themselves into an orgasm, using fantasy, with almost no physical stimulation.

Most men, because they have such limited arousal possibilities compared with women, find the whole subject somewhat fanciful. But women are what I call multi-potential when it comes to sex. Almost anything can arouse some women if the setting, the emotions and the stimulation are right.

stairway to heaven

For both sexes, having an orgasm is rather like walking up stairs. Step by step, increasingly powerful nerve messages accumulate until the sensations reach overload or climax. An initial response in the mind or spirit can be amplified by penis-in-vagina thrusting, a vibrator, and/or rapid hand or finger movements, accompanied by rhythmic contraction of the thigh muscles and much more besides.

Understanding the step-wise nature of orgasms is vital for those women who rarely or never experience them. There are many reasons why this can occur but the most frequent is the lack of reliable, repetitive stimulation that takes them step-by-inevitable-step into overload. Many men get bored or simply don't know how to create a good step-wise build-up, and many women are too shy or don't know how to instruct them. The way most women learn what works for them is through masturbation – which is why it is so useful (see pages 56–9).

oriental insights

Taoist and Tantric theories see orgasm not just as a physiological phenomenon, as we in the West do, but rather as a function of chi or body energy (see pages 12–13).

The testes or ovaries create sexual energies that can either be expelled from the body or recycled within it. 'Outward orgasms' occur only in the genital region and the resulting energy pours outwards from either sex in the form of sexual fluids. It takes a long time to build up this type of energy and a very short time to discharge it. 'Inward orgasms' re-circulate energy through the body's nerves and energy pathways to enliven the whole person, and can, with practice, be extended, not only in time but also in the amount of energy created.

Getting the best out of orgasm, according to Taoist teachings, involves making physical, emotional and spiritual connections with a lover in ways that not only create the maximum possible sexual energy but that re-circulate it within one another's bodies. Fortunately, we don't have to be Taoist adherents to experience the sense of two becoming one in a truly spiritual sex act. But many more Western couples could enjoy soul-to-soul connection during lovemaking if they allowed themselves to focus on shared oneness rather than the ego-centred, goal-seeking sex they usually experience. I hope this book will be of some help on that journey.

his sex organs

the penis

The size, appearance and 'character' of a man's penis are unique to him. Long-term partners or experienced health-care professionals can identify a man by his penis alone, just as podiatrists can identify their patients by their feet.

Men in general can be amazingly uptight about their penis. This is probably not so surprising, given that intercourse isn't possible if a man can't obtain an erection. But it makes almost all men at least somewhat performance-centred, and possibly even performance-anxious. Size is a very common concern, but, unless a penis is very small, most women say they aren't much bothered. Clinical experience shows that most women like a thick penis but aren't too worried about length. In fact, an over-long penis is more of a nuisance than a pleasure for the average woman.

Quite a few of my patients tell me that they are worried in case a new partner thinks badly of their penis or compares it adversely with those of other lovers. Some can't bear to have it seen early on in a relationship. This can make a man unwilling to bare himself for a massage – much to his partner's amazement and frustration.

If you find your man being shy, or worse, about his penis, take time to show him how much you like it. I find that too few women praise their man's penis and many men are too shy to ask if it is OK for her. They act on the fear that it is not. Such men, and they are numerous, may have seen other men's erect organs only in adult videos and assume that they are so poorly endowed their partner will think badly of them or even not want sex with them at all. Of course this is nonsense.

external view

The penis consists of a head (the glans), a shaft and a root (hidden inside the body). If the man hasn't been circumcised, a long, loose tube of skin – the foreskin – covers the glans. This is designed to slide back over the underlying structures, the head and shaft, in a way skin does nowhere else in the body.

The foreskin is a vital part of a man's arousal system – the most important components of erotic stimulation during penile massage or intercourse are sensations from the foreskin itself, a little band of skin called the frenum on the underside of the head, and the glans. And it also contributes greatly to sexual pleasure for both sexes. Because more of the loose skin of the penis of an uncircumcised man remains inside the vagina during sex, the woman's natural lubrication isn't drawn out to evaporate, and this makes sex without additional lubrication more enjoyable.

Clearly, then, the foreskin isn't a useless tube of redundant skin, as many doctors claim. And it should not be removed except in the event of serious medical problems. Yet in the average circumcised man (which is the majority of Americans today), the skin cut away at circumcision represents half the surface area of the whole penis!

internal view

There are three erectile structures inside the penis. When the organ is soft (flaccid), these are like spongy cylinders, but when the man is aroused they fill with blood to become rigid. One of these cylinders sits on the underside of the penis, surrounding the urinary tube (urethra), and terminates as the glans. This is the corpus spongiosum. The other two are located one each side of the upper surface of the penis and are called the corpora cavernosa (singular, corpus cavernosum). About 1cm (½ in) down from the point where the corpora cavernosa join at the penis tip is the male clitoris. This is sensitive mainly to pressure and vibration.

Running through the centre of each corpus cavernosum is one of the two major arteries of the penis. Blood returns from the penis through superficial veins. The corpora cavernosa are rooted in the pelvis, deep in the man's body, creating a strong foundation that prevents the penis from flopping when erect. Surrounding the erectile structures is a layer of connective tissue that holds everything in place and then a final thin layer of skin. Because the two-legged 'root' that anchors the penis to the pelvis is a continuation of the erectile tissues of the penis and eventually connects with the clitoris at the tip of the organ, stroking or rubbing it is immensely pleasurable.

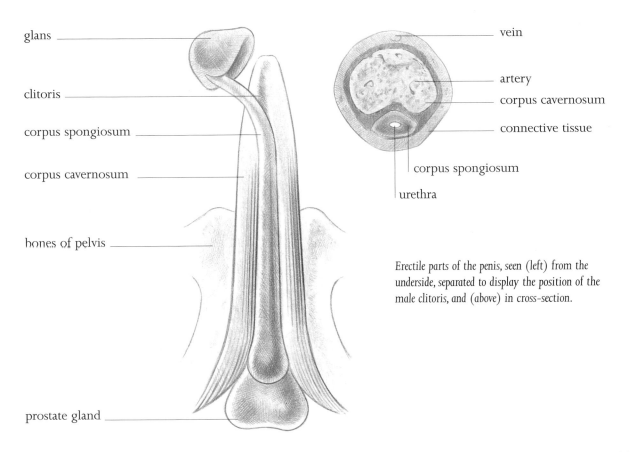

glans

clitoris

corpus spongiosum

corpus cavernosum

bones of pelvis

prostate gland

vein

artery

corpus cavernosum

connective tissue

corpus spongiosum

urethra

Erectile parts of the penis, seen (left) from the underside, separated to display the position of the male clitoris, and (above) in cross-section.

When a man gets sexually excited (physically or mentally), nerve messages are sent to the base of the spinal cord. From here, impulses run to the penis, where they cause the arteries to widen and the veins to contract. This means that more blood flows in than can escape and the penis swells and changes colour.

The brain can contribute positively or negatively to this process. Sexy thoughts can help an erection and various other influences can prevent one. Sometimes the unconscious workings of a man's mind can so affect the nerve pathways that, even if he wants an erection and is getting just the right stimulation, his penis won't respond.

After orgasm, the erection processes reverse and the penis returns to normal. There's usually a short period during which further stimulation will not produce another erection. This can vary from a few minutes in young men to a day in many men over 60. Of course, this varies according to the situation of any individual man.

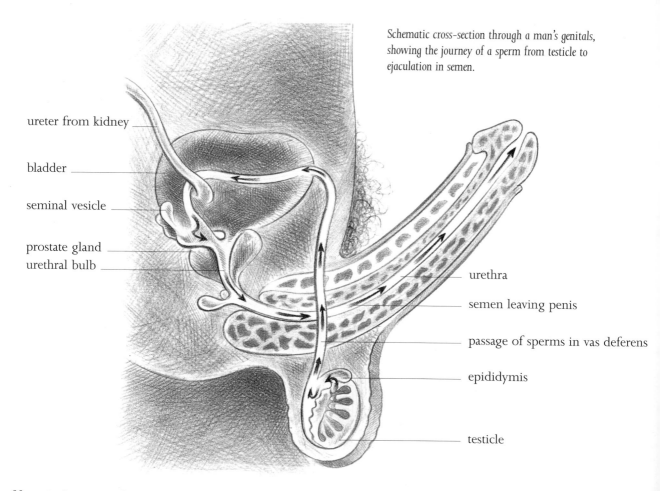

Schematic cross-section through a man's genitals, showing the journey of a sperm from testicle to ejaculation in semen.

ureter from kidney

bladder

seminal vesicle

prostate gland
urethral bulb

urethra

semen leaving penis

passage of sperms in vas deferens

epididymis

testicle

the scrotum and testicles

On the outside of the body, hanging down between the two 'legs' of the penis root, are the testicles, sitting in a bag of wrinkly skin called the scrotum. The position of the testicles is controlled by muscles in the scrotal wall. These can contract, pulling the testicles up towards the body when cold, and relax, letting them down when hot.

Each testis (the medical name for a testicle) is formed of several hundred little lobes, each of which contains highly convoluted tubules storing immature sperms. The testes produce not only sperms but also male hormones. Massaging the testicles has been shown to increase the level of the hormone testosterone in the blood (see testicle and scrotum massage on pages 138–9).

Sperms form and develop in each testicle, later passing into two small organs on top of the testicles called the epididymes (singular, epididymis). Here they mature further and become motile. Then, on each side, they travel along a tube (the vas deferens) that takes them from the scrotum into the abdominal cavity. It is these tubes that are tied when a man has a vasectomy. Sperms are milked as they pass through the vas deferens and then transported to wide areas called ampullae. Later still they are stored in 'bags' called seminal vesicles.

This system means that a man will usually have quite a store of sperms ready to ejaculate, even though any one sperm has taken many weeks to mature. Sperms 'queue up' from the day they are formed until it is their turn to be ejaculated. But when a man comes, the fluid he produces – semen – isn't mainly composed of sperms. It is about 90 per cent prostatic and other fluids produced by the internal sex organs.

the prostate gland and g-spot

The prostate gland sits at the base of the bladder, where the urinary tube exits. It's about the size of a walnut and produces nourishing fluids for sperms as they pass through the tube during ejaculation. The prostate is the site of a man's so-called g-spot. In fact, it's not really a 'spot' at all, but rather the sensitive and sexually arousing parts of the prostate gland. These can be massaged externally (see pages 114–15) or by inserting a finger in the anus (see page 116).

When a man reaches a climax, deep contractions of the pelvic muscles around the seminal vesicles, the prostate gland and the epididymes push sperms and all the fluids produced by the internal sex organs into the first part of the urinary passage (the urethral bulb), where they combine before ejaculation. The pressure of semen passing through the first part of the urinary passage is intensely pleasurable and this, along with rhythmic contractions of the muscles around the prostate gland, is what most men are referring to when they say they have an orgasm.

Many men say their anus and lower rectum are sensitive to sexual arousal. The anus is certainly rich in nerve endings and in blood vessels that swell on arousal (see page 108). These, plus the undoubted psychological thrill of being stimulated in such a 'forbidden' place, make anal play a favourite for many men. Some, consciously or unconsciously, use it as a test of their partner's love for them on the basis that, 'If she'll do that for me, she must really love/fancy me.'

her sex organs

the vulva

In contrast to men, who seem to have a never-ending fascination with their external genitals from babyhood to the grave, most women in Western cultures tend to ignore, or even deny, what's 'down there'. Many never look at their genitals closely and most have no idea how they function in detail. In itself, this hardly matters from day to day but it does amuse me in the consulting room when these same women complain that their guy knows so little about their 'women's bits'.

Like a man's penis, a woman's vulva (the medical name for the external genitals) is as unique as her face. Only a small percentage of women have genitals that look like those we see in books and magazines, and this can be alarming to some. Many women fear that something they come across by chance while showering or during self-stimulation may be a cancer, or some other abnormality. In fact, the overwhelming majority of such fears prove to be ill founded and their genitals are perfectly normal.

Female anatomy certainly makes it harder for women than men to see what their own genitals look like, and because so much more is internal, it can be difficult to know what's what. These pages are designed to accompany personal exploration.

external view, legs slightly apart

If you look at a woman's genitals with her legs slightly parted, only four structures are visible: the mons veneris (the mound covered with hair at the base of her belly), the labia majora (the large or outer lips), the perineum (the area between the vaginal opening and the anus) and the anus itself. The vulva can appear to sit forwards or backwards (towards the anus), according to age and body type. The vulva of a woman with little body fat appears to sit lower than that of a woman with a lot of fat.

The mons veneris is made mainly of fat, probably to cushion the pubic bone during face-to-face intercourse. There are many nerve endings here, and this makes it a great area for massage. The labia majora are two folds of skin that protect and conceal the inner parts of the vulva. These can sometimes be wrinkled like a man's scrotum and, in developmental terms, they originate from the same foetal structures. When a woman is sexually aroused, the large lips swell and become red/pink/brown or even blackish brown. The perineum and anus are both rich in nerve endings and blood vessels, and also respond well to massage (see pages 108–11 and 112–13).

external view, legs wide apart

Once a woman opens her legs widely, other structures become visible. The small lips (labia minora) are the most obvious (see opposite, top). In spite of their name, they may be much larger than the so-called large lips and many women's inner lips protrude outside their large ones. If the inner lips are parted (see opposite, bottom), it's easy to see that they join at the top near the head (glans) of the clitoris. Because the inner lips connect to the hood of the clitoris, vaginal thrusting during intercourse stimulates the clitoral head indirectly. This, plus the sensations of the penis inside the vagina, is what makes intercourse so arousing for a woman.

The glans of the clitoris is partly covered by a small hood, or foreskin. This is continues over and is joined with the skin covering the shaft of the organ. As in a man, the foreskin can be retracted to make the tip more prominent. A short, thin clitoris may have a long, fleshy foreskin; a long, thick clitoris, a short, thin one. The glans is made of erectile tissue like that in the head of the penis.

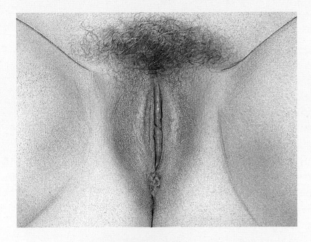

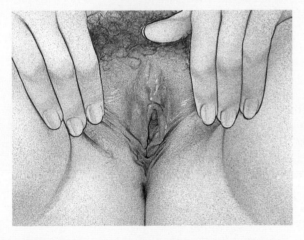

On arousal a woman's glans becomes larger and more sensitive. It remains soft, though, unlike the shaft of the clitoris. The glans is extremely sensitive because it has as many nerve endings as in a man's but in a much smaller area. This is why many women masturbate by stimulating their clitoris indirectly. The shaft of the clitoris can be felt by rolling a fingertip from side to side just above the glans. Most of the rest of the clitoris lies inside a woman's pelvis (see pages 36–7).

Immediately below the clitoris is the opening to the urinary tube (urethra). This is very sensitive to stimulation. Below this lies the vagina. Around its edges may be some small fronds or tags of skin – the remains of the hymen. It can be near impossible to tell whether a woman has ever had intercourse by looking at the remains of her hymen.

the pelvis

The vagina, contrary to popular belief, is a potential opening rather than a gaping cavern. Its walls usually lie flat against one another. It's about 7.5–10cm (3–4in) long but lengthens considerably and balloons at its upper end when the woman is aroused.

Put your finger into the vagina and you'll find it goes backwards and upwards. On the front wall is the g-spot. If you advance your finger deeper still, you'll feel something rigid, about the size of your nose, with a dimple at its centre. This is the cervix – the mouth of the womb (uterus). The cervix enlarges to several times its resting size when aroused.

the reproductive organs

The uterus is a muscular organ about the size and shape of a pear, with its 'pointed' end facing down towards the vaginal opening. The cervix is at an angle to the body of the uterus. Most women experience pleasant sensations in their uterus and cervix when they have an orgasm. Just how much direct stimulation either of these organs can deal with is very personal, with some women literally hating any stimulation and others craving it as their favourite sexual pastime.

On either side of the upper end of the vagina lie the ovaries. They are difficult to feel but sexual hobbyists can usually reach them if determined. Some women enjoy having their ovaries stimulated but most either don't know if they do or actually don't like it once they've experienced it. At the top of the uterus, again at either side, are the fallopian tubes. You can't feel these; they're way too deep inside. Eggs travel down them from the ovaries to the uterus.

the internal clitoris

Over the last few years there have been many important discoveries about the female clitoris. We looked at the 'external' clitoris on page 35. This, we now know, is by far the smallest part of the organ. The whole clitoris is probably bigger than the penis. Imagine a letter Y, turn it upside down and bend the part that now forms the top forward – that is the actual shape of the clitoris. What most people call the clitoris (my 'external clitoris') is really just the tip of this top section.

The 'legs' of the Y extend about 9cm (3½in) into the pelvis and are attached to the pelvic bones. They are just like the 'legs' that form a man's penis root (see pages 30–1) but much larger. In addition to this Y-shaped structure, there are other hidden parts of the clitoris. For example, there are two 'bulbs', one on either side of the vaginal opening, buried within the two large, outer lips.

Another part of the clitoris surrounds the urethra and is known as the urethral sponge. This can be felt in the front vaginal wall as the g-spot (see pages 126–7).

The disadvantage of a fixed clitoris with the vast majority of it beneath the skin is that it offers little freedom for stimulatory movement. Just imagine if the penis were attached to the flesh of the lower abdomen with only the glans free – there'd be no possibility of thrusting in and out. But the advantage of a fixed clitoris is that any downward pull on the foreskin covering the shaft is felt in the glans. So, as a man's penis thrusts in and out of a woman's vagina, it causes indirect stimulation of the glans and sexual excitement, perhaps even to orgasm.

Schematic digrams of the female genitals to show the hidden parts of the clitoris: the three-quarter view (below) and the view from the front (right), showing the smaller 'bulbs' in the outer lips and the larger and deeper 'legs' that attach to the pelvic bone.

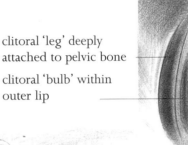

clitoral 'leg' deeply attached to pelvic bone

clitoral 'bulb' within outer lip

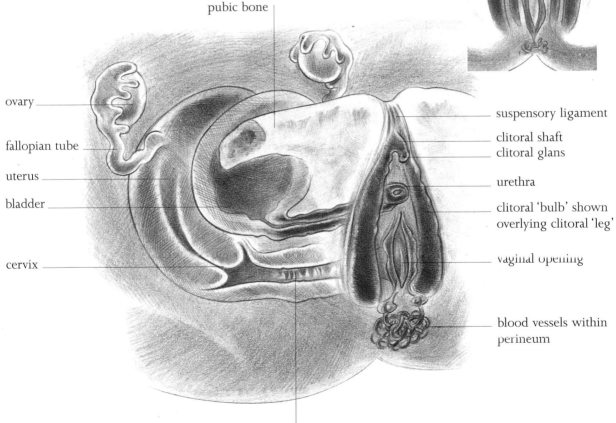

pubic bone

ovary

fallopian tube

uterus

bladder

cervix

vagina

suspensory ligament

clitoral shaft

clitoral glans

urethra

clitoral 'bulb' shown overlying clitoral 'leg'

vaginal opening

blood vessels within perineum

setting the scene

The main thing is to get the 'feel' or mood right. And this will change from day to day, let alone over the years. Of course, you could massage one another out of doors if the temperature is high enough and you can be sure of privacy. And you can do a 'quickie' massage anywhere that feels good. For best results, though, it's worth putting a little thought into your surroundings. They should be romantic, erotic and loving … and getting this right shows how much you care. Here I look at ways to create the best possible environment for an erotic massage session. Page 43 briefly describes the kit you'll need, although you will build up your own collection over time.

soundproofing

I know it's the counsel of perfection but try to design or choose a room that shares few or no walls with spaces occupied by others. If your room has thin walls, think about soundproofing them. You can install sound-insulating board or simply hang heavy rugs. Wood floors are currently very fashionable but they don't deaden sound at all. Quite the contrary, they make it livelier. Put a rug on your floor if this is a problem. To some extent, music can mask some of your lovemaking sounds.

en suite bathroom

Many couples like to bathe or shower together as part of their lead-up to massage. You may also want to bathe or shower afterwards, though towelling down usually removes most of the oil. I know an en suite bathroom isn't possible for many, but it's really great if you have the space. Could you adapt your home?

decoration

Have fun deciding how you want this most intimate space to look and feel. Use the choosing of furniture, fabrics, pictures, and so on to build your loving relationship together. What about some erotic pictures or photos for the walls?

privacy

If you aren't alone in the house, have a lock on the bedroom door. It's hard to relax if you are constantly worried that a child, or someone else, might come in. You could put a Do Not Disturb notice on the door. But this is rather formal, and you'll need to be fairly up-front about your sexual life to do it because it advertises what you're up to. Most lovers massage in the evening, or even just before bed. This can create at least some privacy from the family or other house members but has the disadvantage that you are likely to be tired. One answer for some couples is to take every opportunity to massage one another during the day. It can be a better time to find privacy, and feels deliciously decadent if you're used only to night-time fun.

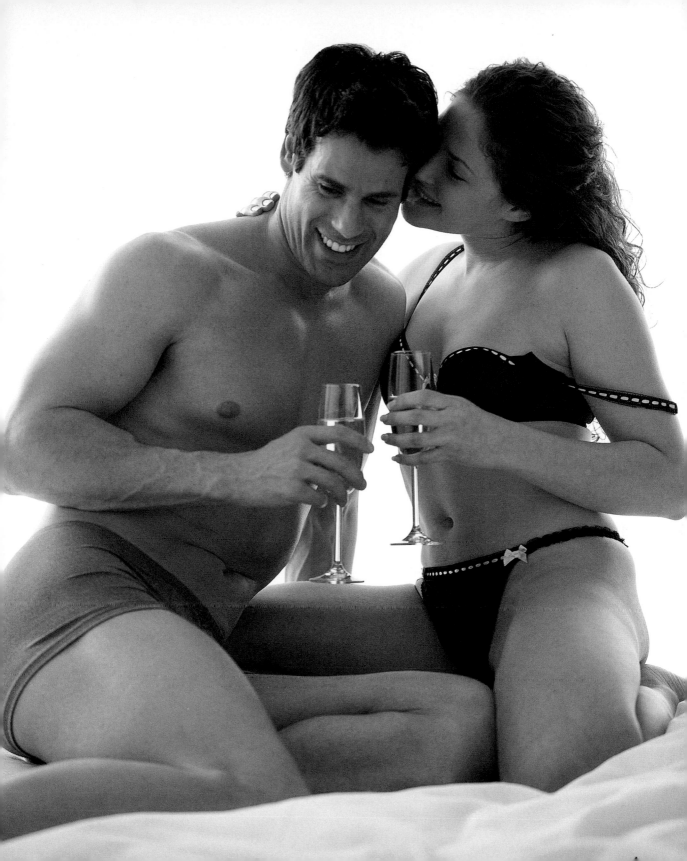

preventing interruptions

The answering machine, if you have one, should be on. Disconnect any other telephones and switch mobiles off. There's nothing worse than that demanding ring just as you're getting in the mood. It can often be near impossible to re-kindle the same feeling, and anyway it's bad bedroom manners as it suggests to your lover that they aren't that important. With cell phones hardly ever switched off, and our virtual addiction to 'noise' of various kinds, it can be a real joy simply to shut out the 'real' world and make ourselves wholeheartedly available for our partner.

lighting

Getting the level right is very important. Harsh overhead lights are no good – install dimmers if possible. If not, cover your bedside lamp with a cloth – taking care not to create a fire hazard – or keep a few low-wattage bulbs handy to replace your usual ones. Candles can be romantic but watch out for safety.

However, when you begin your erotic-massage life together, you'll need quite a lot of light. I've seen many couples where the woman would like to have the place in 'romantic' near-darkness so she can relax – perhaps because she feels ill at ease with her body. But it's not at all romantic to have so little light you can't see and learn from your lover's sexual responses; can't see what you're doing, especially in the genital area, where you need to be quite detailed in your massage; and can't get turned on by watching your partner's enjoyment. I know light level can be a sticky subject for many people but it's worth negotiating on this one. I'm not suggesting you need operating-theatre levels to massage your lover's most sensitive parts accurately and pleasurably but until you are both really skilled it's best to keep the light level fairly high.

Some tell me they don't like being seen while they have an orgasm. I understand their concerns but, if this applies to you, it's worth talking things through and slowly raising the lighting level from near-darkness until you feel comfortable in the light.

heating

In most cool climates this can be the key to a really erotic massage. Couples who don't put enough thought into heating may fail to massage one another at all because the room is always too cold, or rush through a session because they are getting cold. Muscles also tend to respond badly if massaged cold, so a warm room is important.

Central heating is the best answer, of course. Remember to turn it up an hour or so before your session. Many couples keep a small electric fan-heater to boost the temperature quickly for a spontaneous massage. You can also keep your lover covered up where they are not being massaged. Be sure your room is warm but not so hot you're both uncomfortable. I often hear complaints about 'drying out' during a massage session. A large bowl of water will humidify the room and stop sexual lubricants – natural or commercial – from drying out too fast. And it can be nice to keep a glass of water at hand. Massaging can be thirsty work.

private cupboard

Every couple needs somewhere to keep toys and other personal sex 'kit' – such as videos, erotic books and magazines – to prevent them falling into the hands of the children or other members of the household. Ideally, it should be lockable.

mirrors

These can be a sexy addition to your room and make erotic massage really fun – you can see both sides of your lover's body at once. But people react to mirrors very differently so talk this through carefully before getting one. Many women, for example, are horrified to see themselves during lovemaking. Dissatisfaction with their bodies completely spoils the pleasures they would otherwise have. It's probably fair to say that men enjoy mirrors more than women do – mainly, it must be said, to watch their woman, not themselves! A good compromise is to have a tall mirror on a floor stand. This can be angled to show only what you want to see. Ceiling mirrors, much talked and joked about, are probably only for the very few. In all my years working with couples, I have come across only two or three who have actually had one.

TV/video/DVD/PC

If you like to start your session with some sort of erotic relaxation together, you'll need electronics of one kind or another. Although I'd ban TV from the average bedroom on the grounds that it can be abused and actually leads to less sex rather than more, using it for erotic relaxation before a massage session is a very different matter. You could even link your camcorder to the TV and make yourselves the stars of your show, or record your own sexy video for later enjoyment.

music

A CD player set on continuous play is best. Keep the volume low so you can hear one another clearly. Choose gentle pieces, ideally without words. It's hard to concentrate on your feelings, your sensations and your lover if the music is demanding or intrusive. Why not give one another presents of suitable music?

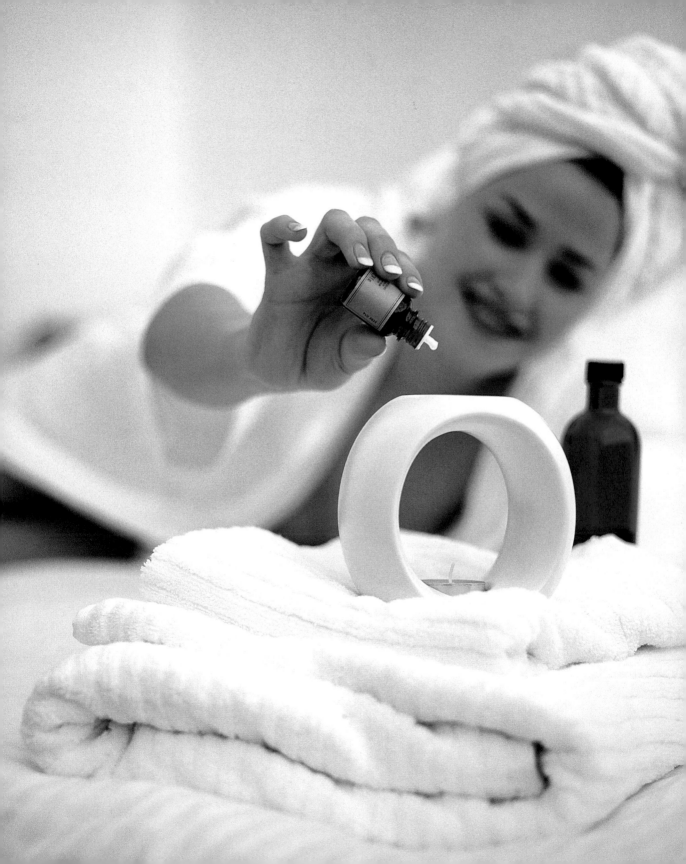

massage kit

What you'll need will depend entirely on how formal your session is going to be and how complicated you want to make it. It's perfectly possible to have a first-class erotic massage session on your bed without any preparation at all. However, some people like to prepare their personal space to make more of an event of their massage. The ideas below are suggestions to set you both thinking about what suits you.

What you'll do will depend on your personalities, your lifestyle, the time you have available that day, what space and facilities you have, and of course how important erotic massage is to you. And you can change things from session to session. On one occasion you might opt for spontaneity, and just have some fun on the bed or in the living room. On another you might go for the whole production and make an evening of it. Preparing can be fun. After all, looking forward to something can greatly enhance its value.

How about taking it in turns to decide what sort of event you want it to be? Send one another a note, email or text message to tease and raise expectations of what's to come.

● **Bed v massage table** Massage tables are only for the really keen. They have the advantage of being the right height, firm and comfortable but are usually too small for anything other than actual massage. The ideal bed is large and firm. Buy the biggest you can afford and that will fit your room. Cover it with a large sheet or something you won't worry about getting oily.

● **Large towels** These will be used to cover those parts of your lover that aren't being massaged at the time.

● **Massage oil** If you want to massage large areas of your lover's body, you'll need some sort of skin lubricant. When it comes to more intimate caresses of the genitals, saliva can be sufficient, though there are purpose-made lubricants (see right). What oil you use, and how you use it, will probably vary from session to session. Anything that pleases you both is acceptable. Vegetable oils such as sunflower, safflower, coconut or olive, all available in your local supermarket, are fine, but there are literally hundreds of sweeter-smelling commercial massage oils available from stores and the net. And you can add a few drops of aromatherapy essential oil if you'd like to increase the erotic mood. Decant enough of your chosen oil for a session into a flip-top bottle so you won't worry about spilling it. Some couples use talcum powder instead of oil. This has the advantage of being 'dry' and non-sticky, but it's not good for genital massage.

● **Sexual lubricant** Water-based ones are fine but dry out and need re-wetting; silicone-based ones are great but last so long on the hands that everything gets covered with them. As with massage oils, there are numerous available commercial variations (see page 117). I don't advise vegetable or aromatherapy oils in the vagina because they can cause infections.

● **Sex toys, especially vibrators** Keep your favourites to hand, ensuring you have enough batteries (see pages 68–71).

● **Clothes** There's no need to wear anything, of course, but some couples say they prefer to be dressed in something that turns the other on. This can be especially important for men, who tend to be more aroused by the sight of a lover dressing sexily.

massage and health

Although most couples who massage one another erotically never come to any harm, it's wise to take some precautions. After all, massage like this is supposed to be healing, sexy and orgasmic. The 'dangers' of erotic massage fall into two broad groups – physical and mental/emotional/spiritual.

physical precautions

As a general rule of thumb, never massage areas where any of the following are present. In fact, it may be possible, even desirable, to massage your lover in certain of these circumstances (if suffering from some forms of cancer, for example) but it's wise to seek medical advice first.

- **Skin conditions** Inflammation of any kind, infectious rashes, boils, sores, bruises or open wounds, burns, bites or stings.
- **Vascular conditions** Very high blood pressure, easily damaged or varicose veins, thrombosis or phlebitis in the legs.
- **Fractures** Within six months of the injury.
- **Disease** Fever, epilepsy, cancer.
- **Undiagnosed** Lumps or tumours, pelvic or genital conditions.
- **Untreated** Sexually transmitted infections.

If you both follow the sequences and suggestions given throughout the book, you will be at little risk of doing one another any harm. But there are several things to avoid, whatever form your erotic massage takes.

● **Direct stimulation over the bony areas of the spine** This is never sexy and can actually be a turn-off.

● **DIY chiropractic** Cracking backs or trying to fix sore muscles or joints is a job for professionals.

● **Heavy pressure in the area of the kidneys in the small of the back** It's unlikely you'll do any harm, but this can be uncomfortable for the receiver.

● **Genital injury** Be sure your partner is highly aroused before genital massage. If they aren't, use plenty of lubrication. If you keep going for a long time, you'll need to refresh water-based lubricants. (Keep a spray bottle filled with water handy.) Be aware that a post-menopausal woman will need a lot more lubrication than a younger one. Short fingernails free from jagged edges are safest; if you have long nails, wear gloves for anal play. Seek medical advice if you are concerned about anything that happens after a session.

● **Sexually transmitted diseases** Opinion varies on how cautious to be about this. As always, if your partner has an active, sexually transmitted infection, you put yourself at risk when you come into contact with their genital secretions or other body fluids. The problem is that it's impossible to know if you have a small cut that could let infections into your bloodstream. So 'safe' massage means being aware, and letting your lover know if there's anything that could put their health at risk. Sadly, people lie about their sex lives – or have been lied to in the past – so neither of you can be sure you know what the truth is.

To be absolutely sure you're safe, use latex or nitrile gloves when in contact with your lover's genital areas or body fluids, including their mouth. When doing a massage that involves only unbroken skin (no body fluids involved), there's no need to wear gloves. Although massage oils and petroleum-based lubricants degrade and eventually destroy latex (which is why they shouldn't be used on condoms), they can be safely used with latex gloves for a short time.

As with any kind of sex play, be sure you never transfer a finger – gloved or not – from a woman's anus (or yours) into her vagina. Doing so can produce some nasty, difficult-to-treat infections.

mental, emotional and spiritual precautions

Looking after, respecting and loving your erotic-massage partner is every bit as important as taking physical care of them and yourself. This level of erotic contact calls for real communication – especially perhaps with a lover you don't know very well. The power for good is huge – but equally harm can be done if you are insensitive, critical, uncaring, deaf to their wishes or acting out, however unconsciously, stuff from your past.

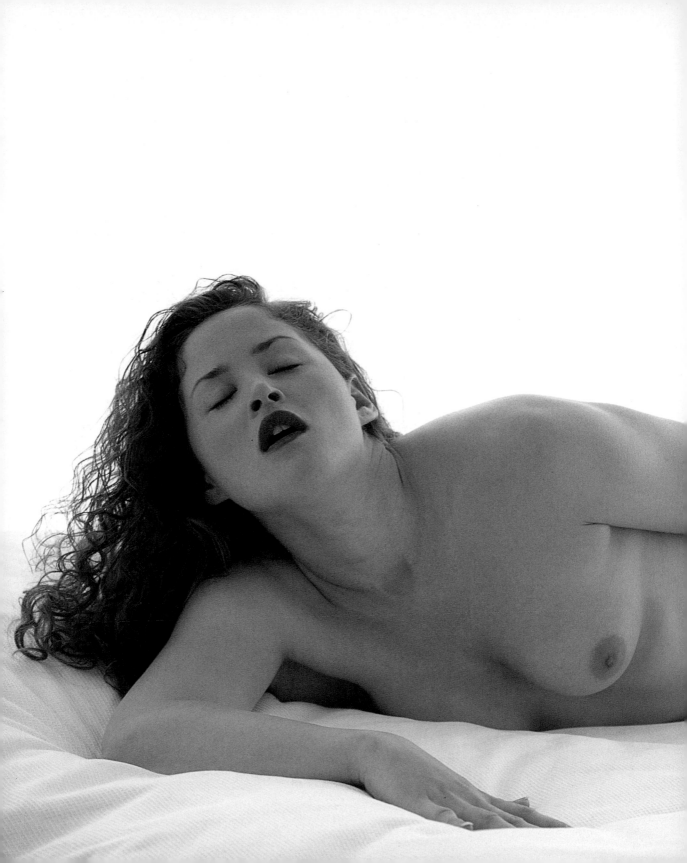

Most of Part One was 'head stuff'. I looked at many of the helpful concepts that it's vital to address if you hope to create an exciting and intimate massage life together. Frankly, without this common ground it's unlikely you'll be on the same wavelength, and so won't enjoy things nearly as much as you could.

part two enhancing your sexual skills

But, between this and the hands-on skills and erotic delights of Part Three, there's a bridge we all need to build if we are to honour our lover and ourselves. This bridge takes the form of learned, practical techniques that prepare us for what is to come.

Erotic massage that's aimed at arousal can be very exciting and a lot of fun. But it can also be a minefield as you unlock feelings, pleasures and emotions you didn't know were there. Because of this, it's essential to become as at ease as you can with your own sexuality, and to be able to control your speed to orgasm, so that when you're engaged in a wonderful, spiritual massage with your lover you're not concerned about, or pressured by, genital relief. Time spent now learning and honing these skills will transform an ordinary massage into a transcendent experience in which you'll experience true intimacy.

introduction

When working with couples on developing their erotic life together, I'm almost always impressed by how little each partner has done to equip him- or herself. In nearly every other area of life we try to obtain the skills necessary to make a hobby or leisure interest more pleasurable and rewarding. Yet few people ever think of doing this in what they claim to be a very important pastime.

I think this is partly a result of laziness and partly because most people see sex as 'natural' – something we 'know about' from some mystical source. Many couples have told me that if they need to work too hard at it then sex can't be right between them. Unfortunately this isn't true.

sex is learned

Research among higher primates shows that almost all sexual behaviour is learned. Young chimps, for example, watch and learn about copulation and then apply their knowledge, often rather ineptly at first, as they become sexually mature. And those who in infancy have no experience of seeing copulating adults are pretty hopeless when they try it themselves.

In modern human communities few of us observe others having sex. This means that unlike our ancestors of only two centuries ago, who lived cheek-by-jowl in large family groupings and shared bedrooms, we have little or no direct experience on which to draw, and as a result are woefully ignorant of what people actually do in bed.

how we learn

Of course, for men and women as for deprived chimps, simple copulation is achievable in time. But few of us want to settle for that. As humans in society, we hope to use sex to create and maintain attachment bonds, to enjoy pleasures at a spiritual and emotional level, and to secure one-to-one man–woman relationships in the interests of raising a family.

So to grow we have to learn from others in some other way. Alas, much of this learning is haphazard, with the emphasis on 'hazard'. Many sexual – indeed relationship – problems arise because of mis-learning … largely from the hard and soft porn industries and their close relative, romantic fiction. I believe we can put this right by making sex an important issue in our lives and by helping one another learn behaviours that are useful and cohesive rather than destructive.

Part Two is about learning to deal respectfully with one's self and with the power that such knowledge brings.

taking responsibility

I've heard so many people claim that their lover should be able to make wonderful things happen for them in the bedroom if they really care for/love/understand them, or whatever. I see things very differently. Each of us has a responsibility to our self, our partner and our relationship to bring as much as possible to the party. Yet time and again the people who complain about what a lover does or does not do in bed have lamentably little self-knowledge to be able to guide a partner. What they are good at is complaining when things don't go as they imagine or fantasize that they should.

I firmly believe that if people can't be bothered to invest in their own sexual empowerment they shouldn't expect others to do their 'homework' for them. If I want to enjoy oil painting as a hobby, I don't expect or demand that my partner teach me everything/get it right for me/make it happen. That would be preposterous.

the route to experience

In Part Two, then, I look at things you can do on your own to build the essential experience you'll need to enjoy erotic massage at a mature, emotional or spiritual level. Imagine yourself a concert pianist. No one wants to listen to you practising a single musical phrase again and again, but once you've mastered the mechanics, your spirit is free to delight us with a performance that comes from the soul rather than the musical score. And it's exactly the same with sex.

There's no better place to start building experience than to learn about your own sexual responses and how to improve them. Self-pleasuring is a vital first step. And I hope that by reading the sections that apply to the opposite sex you'll also gain some insight into what turns them on. Although most people today have several partners before settling down with a special person, this doesn't mean they are all that experienced. They are certainly well versed in their personal experiences but these, it must be said, are often a matter of making the same mistakes time and again. This is hardly experience (or maturity) in any real sense.

Controlling time to orgasm is also a valuable tool. And one best learned alone. Most men in our culture want to delay orgasm while many women want to shorten their time to orgasm. Whatever the wisdom of these aims, the place to learn control is on your own. Then you can offer your skills to your lover as a gift.

But sex isn't just a bodily thing. Simple visualization exercises can help us confront and change attitudes that may prevent us from creating and maintaining a loving understanding through eroticism.

When it comes to sex, you'll never stop learning. You may have your favourite techniques but there are always ways to increase your pleasure and that of your partner. It is because we as individuals are always changing, even after twenty or thirty years together, that we can continue to grow and learn new ways to delight each other.

advantages of self-pleasuring

Masturbation is not the second-best, adolescent pastime that many people, especially men, think it is. In fact, masturbation, or autoeroticism, is the bedrock of great sex with a lover. People who are at ease with their own responses and 'love' themselves make better sex partners because the fantasies, techniques and skills learned during masturbation can enrich their relationships. The couple that get most out of erotic massage have done lots of personal homework first!

There are also many reasons why some people can sustain a good relationship only if they have a rich autoerotic life.

● One partner may want much more sex than the other. Masturbation means the one who wants less isn't pressured or put upon, while the other can maintain their sex drive and interest and still be ready to respond when their lover is in the mood. The alternative is sexual apathy, with resulting disappointment, resentment, bitterness and anger. This is how sex problems start to take root.
● Getting the sort of sex we want with ourselves reduces the hostility that can easily arise if one partner doesn't want a particular sort of sexual activity – perhaps for perfectly sound, if unconscious, reasons.
● If one partner is absent, ill, over-working, stressed, or in any other way sexually unavailable, masturbation comes to the rescue and the relationship is maintained and improved. It is even possible to move things on in your lover's absence.
● Every one-to-one relationship imposes some restrictions on our personal freedom. Autoeroticism helps us retain a sense of freedom and so feel less trapped.

Whatever our feelings about masturbation, and many people even today still feel guilty or ashamed about it, it's not just useful as a way of enriching our relationship – it's good for us as individuals too. And that's no bad thing. After all, our own sexual development doesn't have to stop just because we have a stable sex partnership. Masturbation is helpful and healthy.

● It reminds us that sex is good in itself, partner or no partner.
● It shows we value ourselves enough to produce pleasure that isn't bound up with our relationship and that's important for our emotional well-being.
● It enables us to get things right without involving someone else. Many women say their best orgasms are produced during self-stimulation. For some, masturbation means guaranteed maximum pleasure while still being able to enjoy, or at worst tolerate, sex with their man.
● It's possible to maintain very long periods of near-orgasm and arousal on our own. A lover could get bored, feel left out, used, or possibly even betrayed if we were to behave like this.

- It allows us to indulge our fantasies without interference or distraction.
- Many people have told me they feel bad about engaging in certain fantasies or desires when making love with their partner but that they have no such restrictions or inhibitions when on their own.
- Many people are too shy, ashamed or guilt-ridden to use gadgets, toys, fetish objects, offbeat practices, or whatever, in front of someone else. Autoeroticism involves no such qualms and enables us to be truly ourselves.
- It allows us to distract ourselves from depression, anxiety, and other negative feelings. Of course masturbation is only sticking plaster in these circumstances but that may be all we need from time to time to keep us afloat.

If you had any doubts about it, I hope it's clear how important masturbation is to sexual maturity. 'Real sex' is no more real than masturbation – in fact for many people self-pleasuring is far more real.

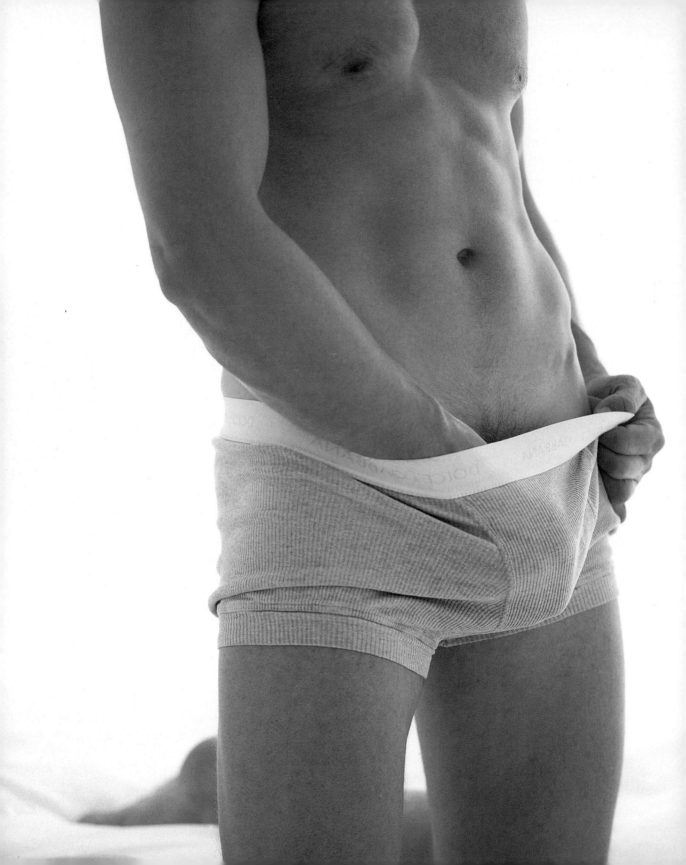

self-pleasuring for him

Most men have never paid much attention to the quality of their arousal and orgasms. Many who became used in adolescence to getting very quickly aroused, and then coming to orgasm very soon after, settle for that level of skill in adulthood. But with training almost every man can increase the pleasure from his erections and orgasms. This involves putting time aside, just as you would for training in a gym, for example, and making yourself the centre of attention. But don't expect instant results. As with any other training, it takes patience and time to get rewards.

improving what you have

The first step to greatly increasing your technique is to use your familiar style of penis stimulation but to enhance it in all sorts of ways. Once you have mastered this, it'll be time to go on to new methods.

Disconnect the phone or turn on the answering machine and give yourself plenty of time. Most men think in terms of a few minutes. I suggest an hour! Get comfortable in a warm room and remove your trousers and underpants. Use some sort of erotic material, or a favourite fantasy, to arouse yourself. Cover your penis liberally with water-based lubricant or scented oil (see page 43). Caress it in your normal way until you get an erection. Now, as you continue to arouse yourself, experiment with getting the very best out of your session by using any of the following suggestions.

● **New positions** If you normally arouse yourself while lying flat on your back, try standing or kneeling, or some other new position. See how different things feel with your legs drawn up to your chest, for example. Take time to experiment.

● **Other parts of your body** Find out how stimulating other parts of your body in lots of new ways can add to your arousal. Stimulate your nipples by applying a clip or clamp or smacking them gently with a light plastic ruler. Play with your scrotum, gently tapping or slapping it. Squeeze your testicles, or pop them between finger and thumb. Press on the area between penis root and anus, checking how it adds to your sensations.

Massage here, using very small, circular motions, and then pat or slap this area. Stroke or massage your anal area, perhaps inserting a well-lubricated finger or butt plug (see page 113) if this appeals.

● **New fantasies** Use erotic literature or videos to top up your fantasy bank. Don't be afraid of things you think others might find perverted. When it comes to arousal, it's vital to banish your internal policeman and simply get on with it. Many men feel stuck with stale fantasies that work just about well enough. Do whatever it takes to produce the highest-quality arousal, even if it feels odd at first.

● **Vibrators** See pages 70–1.

If during any of this you feel like coming, try the squeeze technique (see pages 62–3). Or you can stop and start: do something else for a few minutes and then come back to your training with even a half-erect penis, ready to start over again.

The idea behind this sort of high-quality self-stimulation is to expand your horizons and to become used to taking your time and concentrating on what's going on rather than rushing to orgasm. I know it can be very difficult for some men but try to think of arousal as a journey to be enjoyed rather than a means to an end – ejaculation. Even go without ejaculating at some sessions.

All this practice, perhaps over several weeks, will help you enjoy arousal more, give you confidence you can last for virtually any time you want, and certainly make you a better lover from your partner's point of view. I find that men who learn this sort of control become a lot more confident in and out of the bedroom.

going for it

Now you've improved your arousal and erection quality beyond what you thought possible, it's time for new methods of stimulating your penis.

Most men tell me their current method is perfectly OK and that they can't be bothered to try anything else. This is a pity because most of us are still stuck in that teen-based rut. If you were to suggest that we should do nothing to improve our adolescent attitudes in any other area of life, you'd rightly be ridiculed. Here are some good techniques that are worth trying.

● **Single fist** The standard method, this provides a good, all-round grip and lots of skin-to-skin contact. It also allows you to control the amount of pressure on your most sensitive parts.

● **Fist over fist** Alternate fists, sliding one and then the other from base to tip. A good variation is to use one fist going up and the other going down.

● **Two fists at the same time** If your penis is long enough, this can be fun.

● **Thumb and forefinger** Use your thumb and forefinger, either up and down the whole shaft, or simply up and down the area around the ridge where the head joins the shaft.

● **Both thumbs and forefingers** Make two rings, using the thumb and forefinger of each hand, and place them round your penis. Move both rings up and down in the same or opposite direction, with varying distances between them.

● **Vagina feel-alike** Grasp your penis and squeeze it firmly and rhythmically as your partner would with her pelvic muscles.

● **Foreskin pull** Grasping your penis at about the halfway point, pull down on your foreskin to expose the head. Wrap the other hand around the end of your penis and, with lots of lubrication, stroke up and down the shaft, going almost off the end of your penis and then back down again.

Clitoral 'vibrator' Pressing the pads of the forefinger and thumb of one hand together, pinch the ridge of skin on the underside of your penis head (the frenum) about 2.5cm (1in) from the tip. Now rub your thumb and forefinger together, keeping the hand itself stationary as you vary the pressure and speed. The skin of the frenum should move with the fingertips so that the stimulus happens inside the penis at the clitoris.

Split fingers With the fourth and fifth fingers of one hand on one side of the shaft and the second and third fingers on the other, massage your penis using lots of lubrication. Now massage your scrotum and testicles at the same time with your free hand.

The pump Lie down on your back with your knees bent and pointing outwards so that the bottoms of your feet are touching. As you ejaculate, bring your knees almost together and then back out again in a pumping action. Keep on pumping until you stop spurting semen.

Slapping or beating With your penis between your palms, use both hands at once, or slap it against your stomach. You can even beat it against another object.

Foreskin massage Pull your foreskin all the way back and lubricate the penile shaft. Now rub up and down it, pulling and stretching at the same time. This can produce very 'sharp', almost painful sensations ... and an excellent orgasm.

The screw Lubricate your erect penis very well. Grasp it in a reverse hold so your thumb is pointing down towards the base and move your whole hand up and down in a screwing and unscrewing motion, gripping firmly all the time. This provides a range of novel sensations, even for the sexually experienced man.

Tiptop Masturbate with one hand in your normal way but hold the palm of your free hand just above your penis head so at each upward stroke you strike the palm gently but firmly.

Pillow play Place a pillow under your belly and lie face downwards, thrusting between the pillow and the sheets.

Insertion There are many objects into which you can insert your penis to mimic a vagina – watermelons, cardboard toilet-roll inners, purpose-made sex toys, penis pumps, and much more. Use your imagination but be careful.

Water delights Direct the spray of a shower on to your penis head. If your shower is pumped, you'll find the sensation exceptionally arousing when your foreskin is drawn back. Take the head off the shower too, and experiment using the powerful stream of water.

self-pleasuring for her

It's easy to get lazy about arousal over the years – to settle for the minimum you can get away with. A number of women I've treated believe, at some unconscious level, that they don't deserve really high-quality orgasms. Some don't have orgasms at all. Perhaps they are guilty about sex, afraid of it, can't be bothered or are too tired to go beyond the minimal pleasure they experience, fear a partner's response if they were suddenly to become demanding sex goddesses, and so on. The reasons are numerous. Some even unconsciously punish a lover by having poor orgasms, perhaps because he is unrewarding, inconsiderate, critical or unloving out of the bedroom.

Most women can teach themselves to have better-quality, more numerous or quicker orgasms if they are prepared to take time training. And sex with a partner can be greatly improved the more expert you are on your own arousal. The first step to increasing your self-stimulation skills is to enhance what you'd normally do. When you're confident that you can have much more rewarding orgasms, it'll be time to introduce new stimulation methods.

improving what you have

Feeling really relaxed and safe is probably even more important for a woman's arousal than it is for a man's. Organize things so you'll have an hour or so to yourself. Many women I see set aside 10 minutes and then wonder why they don't get much out of the session.

Make sure the room is warm, the phone unlikely to disturb you, and maybe even light some candles. Have a bath or shower beforehand if it helps. Ensure the lighting is right – not so dim you can't see but not so bright it's intimidating. Have a small alcoholic drink if that works for you. Relax with an erotic video, romantic novel, or whatever turns you on.

Taking time to set the scene like this is very important. Some women who find erotic massage hard tell me they simply don't spend much time pleasuring themselves, let alone encouraging their lover to pleasure them. Sensual preparation will help you realize how important you are – how much you deserve delightful sensations and pleasures. And this is the foundation for really enjoying an erotic massage with your man. So many women today are rushed all the time. Stressed and trying to do too much, they forget how to turn off and get turned on!

● **Getting started** Lie naked on the bed or sofa and caress your whole body with talc. It's less messy than oil. Orgasm isn't the goal here – pleasure is.

● **Looking and feeling** Placing a small hand mirror between your legs, find a comfortable position in which you can see your genitals. Caress yourself as you look in the mirror, linking what you see with what you feel. Put a finger inside and see how wet you are. Learn to recognize how your aroused body feels and then to link this to how wet you are. More wetness means higher arousal.

● **Masturbating** Stimulate yourself in any familiar way you find pleasurable, getting increasingly specific about exactly what excites you best.

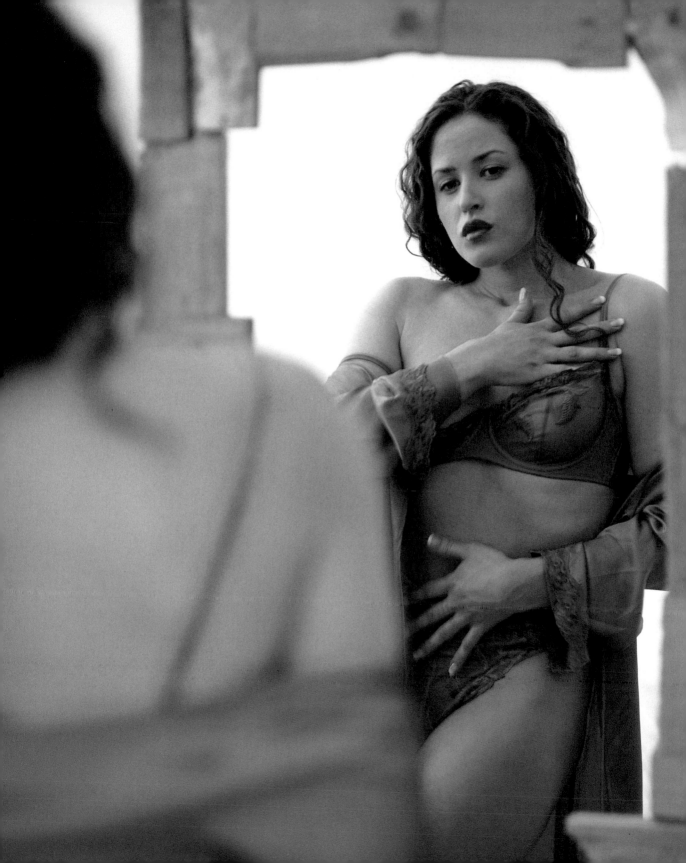

Such exploration will help when your lover pays attention to your genitals. Some women say they hardly know themselves at all, and clearly find it very difficult to guide a lover to what's best for them. Others hand responsibility for their arousal over to a lover and then get annoyed when he doesn't produce magic sensations for them. This is neither fair nor loving.

Working with women over the years has taught me how difficult many find it to know how aroused they are. A man's penis is a pretty obvious arousal meter. A woman's wetness – the equivalent of an erection – is far subtler!

And some women find it hard even to recognize how they feel inside — I have seen women who can have an orgasm and not know it.

A method I've used in such circumstances involves scoring on a scale of 1 to 5 how aroused you think you are. Start your stroking or caressing a long way away from your genitals, rating your response at each body area, and actually record the results on a sheet of paper. Several parts of your body might make you feel like coming when stimulated. Note that on your score sheet too. And when masturbating, use the same scoring system until you can increase your scores to near 5 every time, whatever you are doing.

At first this will all seem rather pathetic but over the weeks you'll notice how much more accurate your scoring becomes. This method seems to make pleasure more likely because it takes everything out of the woolly realms of 'sensation' into something more immediate, quantifiable and 'real'.

going for it

Most women have a favourite way of caressing their clitoris for maximum effect. This doesn't, however, mean it can't be improved on. Some women, for example, have never put fingers inside themselves at the same time. Others have never used a dildo or butt plug along with clitoral stimulation. Many women have never explored the potential of greater nipple stimulation while they masturbate. And so on.

Try any familiar and effective stimulation techniques in combination. And then experiment with the suggestions below.

One real problem women complain to me about is running out of hands! Set your mind to ways of solving this. Nipple clamps, for example, keep themselves in place. Wear a pair of panties to secure a dildo or butt plug — or both! — so as to leave your hands free for your clitoris, or whatever. Be creative.

● **Water delights** Bathtub taps, showerheads (especially those that 'massage'), and even Jacuzzi jets can all produce great sensations if used creatively. Jacuzzi play must be done with care. Never get too close to the jets as they can force water or air into your vagina and that can be dangerous. And before you begin any water play, test the temperature, avoiding very hot water. In a bathtub about half full of water, sit with your vulva directly underneath the taps and use one hand to open your lips so the water can trickle directly on to your clitoris. You can try this with hips tilted upwards too. Remove the showerhead and direct the water flow on to your clitoris. Obviously, the faster it is the more stimulation, but some women like to arrange the flow to just drip or drizzle.

● **Proprietary sex toys** Mail-order catalogues and adult stores have literally thousands of different toys on offer. Experiment with vibrators, dildos, anal toys, nipple pleasers, and so on. Do anything that increases your level of arousal or orgasm quality.

● **Household objects** I'm not a great fan of these because they are often dangerous — they can break or hurt and cannot easily be cleaned. But, whatever I think, women will continue to pleasure themselves with hairbrush handles, candles, vegetables, washing machines set to spin, and much, much more. As women become less inhibited about buying toys made for the purpose, these makeshifts will slowly become redundant.

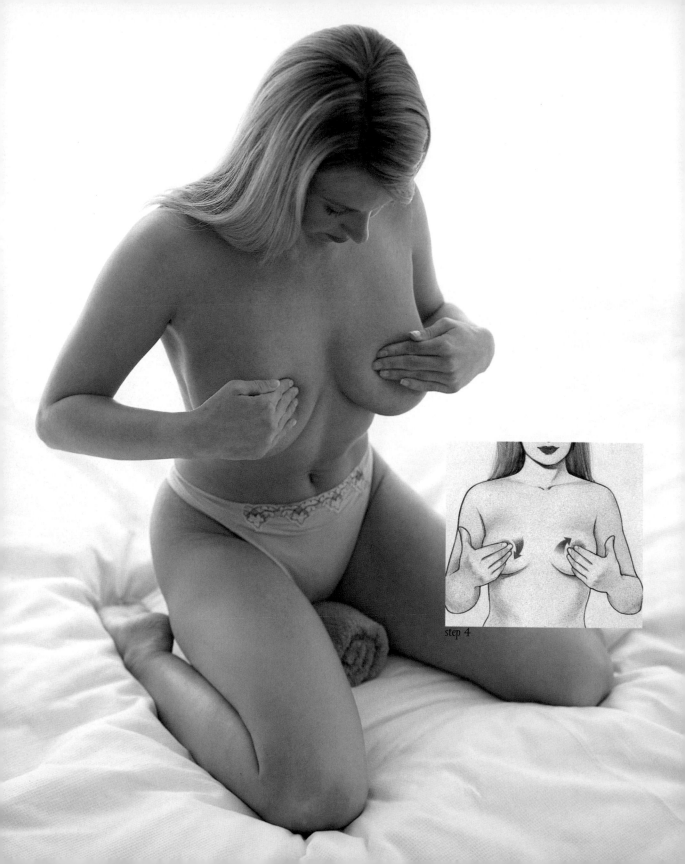

step 4

enhancing sexual energy

With this delightful, erotic breast massage a woman can enhance her sexual energy in a healing, spiritual, self-loving way. You could try it on its own, use it as a prelude to self-pleasuring, or make it a part of your preparation for an erotic massage with your partner. According to ancient Taoist principles, breast massage like this activates energy not just in your genitals but also in many of the body's vital glands. By the end of this exercise you should be feeling relaxed, aroused, energized and ready for anything.

Sit on, or kneel over, a fairly hard, round object, such as a rolled-up face flannel or a soft ball, to put pressure on your genitals. Cover your breasts with talcum powder, if you want to stay dry, or fragrant massage oil, if you want lubrication.

1 Imagine you are drawing sexual energy all the way up from the very base of your spine to your head. Try to focus it in the centre of your forehead between your eyes.

2 When you can do this confidently, try re-directing this spine-based energy to your nipples. Visualize it flowing into your breasts and creating warmth in your nipples.

3 Rub the palms of your hands together to create warmth and energy and then place them on your breasts, feeling the heat. Press your tongue firmly up against the roof of your mouth. Close your eyes and breathe deeply.

4 Massage your breasts, using the second, third and fourth fingertips of both hands as pads in a small, circular action as you gently press the breast tissue against your ribcage. Maintain constant contact with your skin as you work your way round your breasts, moving one hand clockwise and the other anti-clockwise, to finish with your fingertips at the base of the breastbone.

5 Place the second joint of the middle finger of each hand directly on the nearest nipple, allowing the rest of each hand to lie flat and pointing inwards. Your fingertips are now resting about 4cm (1½ in) from the nipples. Massage here with tiny, circular motions (again the same hand clockwise and the other anti-clockwise). This, according to Taoist theory, stimulates the endocrine glands throughout the body.

6 Repeat the massage described in step 5 through all the remaining steps, as you focus on your feelings and breast sensations. You should soon begin to sense your clitoris getting aroused, and you may also feel some pressure in your forehead as sexual energy builds up.

7 Concentrate on your breathing and try to channel the energy this produces into your breasts. This will take some practice.

8 Contract and release your pelvic-floor muscles repeatedly, focusing on the ever-increasing sensations in your vagina.

9 Channel your breath energy into your vagina, your vulva and all your pelvic organs.

10 Imagine your nipples, clitoris and vagina all joined by a magic thread. Starting at the base of your spine, draw your energy from here up to your forehead. When it is very obviously there, take it down to your nipples. Focus on the sensations in them. Then take the energy down to your clitoris and feel it getting warm. Finally, take the energy into your vagina, feeling it getting very wet.

controlling time to ejaculation

Most men say they'd like to last longer. This is especially true of younger men, who tend to come very quickly in their 'trigger-happy' years. There are many reasons why a man may ejaculate before he wants to: early adverse sexual experiences, performance anxiety, lack of awareness of the internal cues the body gives, and, paradoxically, low arousal level or sex drive. Of course each man has his own definition of what 'premature' means. I've had patients complain because they can't hold off for an hour – and others because they come before they have an erection!

Before starting on any sort of self-help, it's vital to know your body and its responses in some detail. There comes a point when no man can hold back. To be able to control your orgasm, you need to be aware of what's happening at this point – and, more importantly, just before it. This is where the stop–start can help. When you need only one or two stops during a 15-minute session, you're ready to move on to the squeeze. But be patient – stop–start could take some weeks, or longer, to get right.

Once you have mastered the squeeze, ask your partner to arouse you and teach her how to do it too. She should become as expert as you are. One day, ask her to get on top of your erection. She shouldn't move at all. At subsequent sessions, ask her to move more and more until you can last a long time. If you feel like coming, she can jump off, do the squeeze to calm you down, and then repeat the process.

the stop–start

1 With a dry hand, try to masturbate for 15 minutes without ejaculating. Be very aware how aroused you are: if it helps, create a personal rating scale (see page 23) and be able to tell yourself where you are on it at any moment.

2 When you feel you are about to come, stop all stimulation, focus on exactly how you feel in your genitals and take some very deep breaths. Let your arousal level drop for a little while and resume only when you feel that you are ready for excitement.

3 Repeat this cycle several times until you can last for 15 minutes.

4 Do the same thing, but now with lubricant. This is much more arousing and, as a result, more difficult to control. Start with small, slow movements, increasing the amount of stimulation as you gain in confidence.

the squeeze

1 With a dry hand, masturbate to the point when you know from experience that you're about to come.

2 Take the head of your penis between the fingers and thumb of one hand and squeeze hard just below the rim. This will make your erection subside quickly.

3 Repeat the cycle several times, focusing each time on the many exciting sensations of arousal deep inside your pelvis.

4 Repeat, using lots of lubricant, until you can last as long as you want at any session.

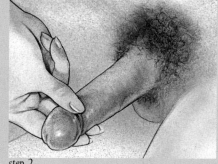

step 2

There are several tricks worth trying when making love with your partner, if you want to be able to repeat your practice level of control over time to ejaculation. Here are the two most helpful ones.

● **Alter thrusting.** Slow the tempo of thrusting, and experiment with changes of angle and depth. Very deep penetration may be best because the head of your penis will be less stimulated by your partner's ballooned vagina.

● **Think yourself out of it.** Some men find it helps to talk through an internal 'script' that slows them down. Or to take time out before sex to imagine doing it really well. Visualization (see pages 66–7) is useful here. Imagine entering your partner, feeling relaxed and comfortable, and just being still in her vagina. Now imagine thrusting very slowly. Then increase the power of your thrusts. Slow down again. Next, increase your thrusting until you feel excited. Slow down and focus on feeling calm and happy. Eventually, let yourself come and tell yourself this is how it will be in reality. It can also help to focus on parts of your body other than the genitals. Most men get over-involved with their genitals during these exercises.

If premature ejaculation is a problem, creating or restoring good communication between you and your partner will help enormously (see pages 20–3). Don't have intercourse for a while – go back to courtship behaviour. Whatever you do on your own, when you do resume lovemaking, focus together more on other parts of your body – almost all premature ejaculators become obsessed with their genitals – and learn to become somewhat passive as she helps you overcome the difficulty.

controlling time to orgasm for her

Many women have problems with orgasm. Some take a very long time to come – they may even give up, dispirited, when things don't happen quickly enough – and others find their orgasms are over too soon to enjoy. A substantial minority are in the habit of faking it when with a man. Unfortunately, there are many impediments in the way of good orgasms – far more than in men. The most significant are listed below.

● **Physical** Diabetes; hormonal deficiencies; fear of becoming pregnant or, paradoxically, not getting pregnant.

● **Psychological** Inability to relax; fear of criticism or loss of control; unconsciously seeing her partner as a father; unconsciously identifying with a (sexless) mother; childhood conditioning that sex was 'bad' or sinful; depression; anorexia; feeling mutilated after surgery (for example, a hysterectomy); latent lesbian thoughts in heterosexual women.

● **Emotional** Falling out of love; during an affair due to feelings of guilt or shame.

● **Sexual** Poor masturbation methods; unwillingness or inability to experiment; unimaginative, inexperienced or off-putting lover who may also be selfish.

Any of these impediments can prevent a woman having orgasms at all, or having enjoyable ones. Many benefit from professional help. Some, though, can be remedied using this book. Taking time to make an investment in your erotic life can turn around even some quite serious conditions. You could be surprised how much progress you can make, either alone or with your partner's help.

helping yourself

Be honest. Many women I see fool themselves, or their men, and then wonder why they don't get the result they want. This is no time to pretend, hoping that your partner will somehow know how to 'rescue' you from your arousal problems. And I'm not just talking about faked orgasms – though they are dangerous enough – I mean pretending to yourself that things are better than they are, perhaps to keep the peace.

Talk things through with your partner. He should be your best friend and helper in your journey. Try to discover between you what's going on and how you could improve matters. Your partner may be able to help not only with your relationship – because he's a part of it – but with insights into your personal sexuality – because he knows you so well. A loving partner who wants the best for you can be a formidable ally.

See a doctor. This is a priority if you think ill health or medications could be causing your arousal problems.

Learn about your genitals. See pages 34–7. An important starting point.

Spend much more time masturbating. See pages 56–9.

Try to improve your fantasy life. Read erotic literature, watch sexy videos, write an XXX-rated video script yourself, and so on. If you can, share your fantasies with your lover, asking him to talk you through them while you do erotic things together. You might even want to act out a fantasy, but go carefully with this one.

Tell your partner how he can help. Many women who endure poor stimulation from their men find that the longer they leave things un-said, the more difficult it becomes to raise the issue. Don't attack him or criticize his poor technique. Rather praise him when he gets things right and gently guide him to what's best for you.

Use visualization. It's an effective way to improve arousal (see pages 66–7).

Get your pelvic muscles into shape. See pages 72–3.

Get a good vibrator and use it! See pages 68–9.

Listen to other women's experiences. Some of my patients say they've found real value in doing this. Of course, it's only useful with people you can trust, and they have to have something to say.

visualization

Think about what happens to your body as you watch a really exciting film in the cinema. The changes are very much like those that would occur if the events were happening for real. In other words, our bodies can be tricked into believing in a reality that's in fact is only 'real' in our minds.

In my work with patients I use this psychological trick a lot. And it's a very powerful one. Over thirty years ago psychologists found that cancer sufferers who imagined their white blood cells destroying their cancer cells survived twice as long as patients who didn't employ this sort of visualization.

In the sexual life, visualization can be used to help achieve many of the results you want. If you come too fast or too slowly, are ill at ease with your body, are shy or guilty about something to do with sex, are afraid of sex, need help building sexual arousal, or if you are going off your partner, then visualization can really help. The key is to practise every day, perhaps for some weeks, making your scene increasingly rich in detail and positive experiences.

Rather like a fantasy, visualization is a mental game in which you imagine a scene or situation. The secret of success is to employ all your senses to create the scene in your mind's eye. I usually start by asking people to imagine themselves on a beach. However nice this might be, they get really good results only when they can taste the salt in the air, smell the seaweed, hear the children playing, and feel the warmth of the sun. Only then is it possible for their minds to convince them that they are actually at a beach – not just thinking about one or imagining it in their mind's eye.

1 Work out a really sexy storyline that achieves the end-result you want, remembering to include experiences, sensations and events for all your senses.

2 Write the whole story down, making the main character an idealized 'you'. If you write a tale that embodies all your real-life neuroses, worries, failings and so on, you'll get nowhere. Record the whole thing on tape if you like, reading it slowly and in a very relaxing voice so it's nice and easy to listen to time after time, perhaps over some weeks.

3 Go somewhere quiet where you won't be disturbed and lie down, or sit in a really comfortable chair.

4 Breathe slowly and deeply for a minute or two until you feel pleasantly relaxed, keeping your eyes closed throughout. Try to empty your mind. This takes some practice.

5 Starting at the top of your head and working right down to your feet, actively contract and relax each group of muscles in turn. Feel the tension leave each area before going on to the next. Once you've worked on your feet, your whole body should feel warm, relaxed and rather heavy.

6 Think through your story in your mind's eye or listen to your tape, getting deeply into the feelings. You could be surprised how your body reacts. You may, for example, actually become aroused.

7 At the end, keep your eyes closed, remain seated or lying down, and relax into the pleasant feelings for a few minutes.

This whole session might take about 10 minutes. Repeat once a day, ideally. You can do it anywhere once you get into the habit. I have patients who do it while waiting for their kids to come out of school, on a train, or even at the dentist! Over time you may find you need, or want, to change the imagery. This can also be a good way of training yourself to deal with new situations in your sexual life.

vibrators for him

Few men think of using a vibrator on themselves. And even fewer of their partners think of doing so. This could be because the range of sexual thrills a vibrator can produce for a man is much smaller than that for a woman. But this doesn't mean it's not worth trying. Unfortunately, many men see vibrators as 'women's toys' and so feel less than manly even wanting to experiment. This is a pity because they miss out on two great pleasures.

Although a few men say they are turned on by vibrating their testicles, perineum or anus, clinical experience tells me there are only two places that men find vibrator stimulation really exciting – their clitoris and their g-spot. Unfortunately many men don't know where these are! (For advice on vibrator care, see page 68.)

stimulating your clitoris

We saw on page 31 that a man has a clitoris. It is situated deep in the head of the penis – underneath the little fold of skin on the underside. Though the male clitoris can't be seen, it is – as for a woman – a very potent source of sexual pleasure. Some couples discover it accidentally as they learn how arousing it is when the woman vibrates her fingertip over this area.

One day when you are aroused, take time to find your clitoris. Pull your foreskin (if you have one) back and lubricate the area over and around the little vertical fold, or frenum, on the underside of the head. Press deeply into the fold, sensing how it feels, and sandwich the clitoris within between your forefinger and thumb. Gently roll your forefinger over it until you find a pleasurable sensation. Now gently tap the area repeatedly. Then press your fingertip deeply into your penis over the clitoral area and vibrate it, perhaps for some time.

Stimulation of the clitoris can result in ejaculation without erection. It's an important lesson for the average Western male. We are brought up to believe that a man can have an orgasm or ejaculate (and these are different things) only if he has an erection. This isn't the case. A man can experience three different types of genital arousal – erection, ejaculation and orgasm – and they do not have to go together. It is possible to have an erection and not ejaculate or have an orgasm; to have an orgasm without being erect or ejaculating; and to ejaculate without an erection or orgasm. Understanding this and experiencing it can completely turn around your attitude to arousal in erotic massage.

If you use a vibrator that produces deep waves of sensation rather than a shallow buzz, you'll experience some very pleasant feelings within 10 seconds. Many men can have an orgasm or ejaculate with this sort of stimulation. The sensations are very different from those experienced with normal penile stimulation.

1 Lie down or sit comfortably with your genital area exposed and lubricate the head of your penis well. It isn't necessary to get an erection. You'll see why in a moment.

2 Lay your penis flat on your lower belly and apply the vibrator to the little vertical fold of skin. Press quite firmly

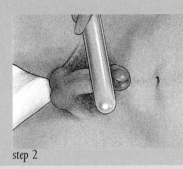
step 2

downwards, trapping your penis head between your belly and the vibrator.

3 Try various pressures, focusing on the different sensations, until you discover what is best for you. Eventually you'll ejaculate without manual stimulation, perhaps even with only a partial erection – or with none at all.

stimulating your g-spot

Using a g-spot vibrator, it's possible to reach your prostate gland (see pages 32–3) and stimulate it very effectively. You can ring changes on the basic method below. Once you've hit the spot, try moving the tip as it vibrates to massage the prostate or stimulate your penis while vibrating your g-spot. It might take a little time to find just the right places.

1 Find a comfortable position – lie down with your legs pulled back, or squat on your haunches – and arouse yourself.

2 Once you have a good erection, lubricate your anus generously and insert a finger or two to open it up a little.

3 Lubricate your g-spot vibrator and insert it slowly, pushing the tip forwards as you aim for your navel. If you are new to anal insertion, this action will be very different from putting an object into your partner's vagina. The vagina goes downwards and backwards. The anal canal goes upwards and forwards.

4 Experiment with positions until the tip gives the sensations you want. Don't be surprised if you have an orgasm or ejaculate without an erection, or only a partial one.

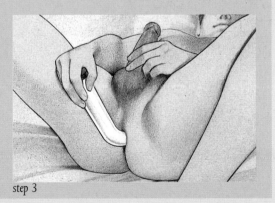
step 3

pelvic-muscle training

Many of the great sensations we experience during high arousal and orgasm are produced by contractions of the muscles in the pelvis. In a man, these muscles lie at the root of the penis and around the anus, and in a woman they form a figure-of-eight around the vaginal and anal openings.

Like any other muscles in the body, they become flabby and unfit if not used and benefit from training. But strengthening them isn't just an end in itself. Well-toned pelvic muscles can greatly help women who develop a floppy, unresponsive vagina after childbirth or the menopause, and those with poor bladder control. A man who is losing his erective power can also benefit from strengthening his pelvic muscles.

Some women find that doing pelvic exercises (also known as Kegels) enables them to have multiple orgasms for the first time. And, even more significantly, many women report that learning pelvic-muscle control helps them get more pleasure out of penile penetration, while hugely increasing the pleasure their men feel as the penis is 'milked'. Some women can actually bring a man to orgasm by this milking alone – he doesn't need to thrust.

The exercises that follow are for both sexes. Don't attempt the second until you have mastered the first, and so on.

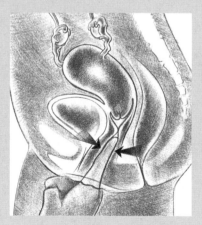

● **Contractions** Wait until your bladder is full. While peeing, contract your pelvic muscles to stop the stream. Don't use your abdominals. Improve this control day by day until you can stop and start peeing at will.

● **The elevator** You need an empty bladder for this one. Imagine your pelvis to be an elevator and, starting at the ground floor, take it slowly up to the fifth. Over some weeks' practice you should be able to take your elevator to any floor and hold it there.

● **The flutter** Any time, any place, tense your pelvic muscles and flutter them ten or twenty times. Repeat several times a day.

There are several ways to check progress. A woman can insert a finger into her vagina (see above) and try to trap it there by contracting her muscles. A man can do the same with his anus, but it's rather more difficult to achieve. A woman with very strong muscles should be able to clamp them so hard on a pencil (blunt end inside!) that it's almost impossible to withdraw it. I don't advise this is as a test for men.

only for the advanced

The final stage of pelvic-muscle building is
weight training. This exercise was devised for
women but it is also suitable for men. You may
find it creates some exciting and novel sensations
in your pelvis or even elsewhere.

You need a stone or wooden egg with an
'eye' fixed to the pointed end (see page 74). On
this you will hang a series of weights. If you
don't have weights with hooks to attach to the
eye, find a small, light bag to contain them.
Once you're fully aroused, insert the egg, wide
end first, into the vagina (or anus, for men).
Begin with a weight of about 250g (9oz) and
let it hang there as you grasp the egg with your
pelvic muscles. Over time you'll be able to
increase the weight. It's unwise to exceed about
3kg (6½lbs). Be guided by common sense.

You'll find it easier to start with a fairly
large egg. Decrease the egg size as your pelvic
muscles become very strong. Real experts can
swing a heavy weight on a small egg and still
keep the egg firmly in place.

strengthening your vagina

Doing regular pelvic-muscle exercises (see pages 72–3) will strengthen your vagina. But there's another effective technique that originated in ancient China and involves a solid egg placed in the vagina.

You can look on the net for suppliers of ready-to-go wooden or stone eggs. Choose one about 2.5cm (1in) in diameter. The smaller the egg the more work your vaginal muscles have to do. Some women start with a much larger egg and graduate to a smaller one. The egg must have a strong cord attached to its pointed end. Clean your egg thoroughly before you use it for the first time: boil it in water or soak it in disinfectant for an hour. After use, just wash it in warm water.

It is vital to get your sex hormones energized before starting egg exercises. So spend at least 5 minutes massaging your breasts deeply. Begin near the nipples and work outwards to cover both breasts. You'll know you're having the right effect if your nipples harden and your breasts feel fuller. Then spend at least another 5 minutes stimulating your clitoris and outer vulva until you are highly aroused.

It helps to know about the different zones of the vaginal canal before inserting the egg. I ask my patients to visualize these sections as if they were parts of an elevator shaft. It's easier, then, to imagine exactly where the elevator is at any time. This makes you more aware of what's happening in your vagina and that, in turn, will enable you to use your vaginal muscles better during lovemaking.

The first section of the vaginal canal includes the muscles around the external opening and the lowest part of the canal. The third section is high up, right next to your cervix, and the second section is in between. Many different muscles surround the second and third sections, all of which can be used to move your egg in various directions. This will sound somewhat fanciful if you've never tried it. But with practice you'll see what I mean.

The very act of trying to learn this degree of pelvic-muscle control and awareness is a great start. Few women are aware of just how much is going on in their pelvis. Or more to the point, how much more could happen, given some dedication.

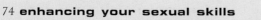

While I accept that this kind of detailed interest isn't for every woman, all those whom I know that have made an effort to get to understand themselves in this way have had nothing but delight from the experience. To far too many women the vagina is some sort of 'black hole' into which things, including their lover's penis, disappear in some mystical way. The notion that it is a highly dynamic space that can be actively used to enhance their and their partner's enjoyment comes as news to most of them. Egg exercises are a good start on this journey of discovery.

1 When you are aroused (breast and genital massage done, see text opposite), insert your egg, wide end first.

2 Adopt the yoga Horse Stance (see illustation opposite) and contract the first section of your vagina to help keep the egg securely in place.

3 Inhale deeply and contract the muscles at the very top of your vagina. This, in fact, contracts sections two and three simultaneously, moving the egg upwards into the second section. You'll feel it moving.

4 Squeeze the egg lightly with the second section, getting a good grip on it. This takes some practice.

5 Try to move the egg slowly up and down the vaginal canal. You'll have to use your mind as well as your muscle contractions to shift it. When you are out of breath, rest. You'll feel energy building up inside your pelvis.

6 Experiment with moving the egg sideways. Again, this takes practice. Once you have the knack, you should be able to move the egg sideways and up and down at will. As you become more skilled, vary both the speed and power of your contractions.

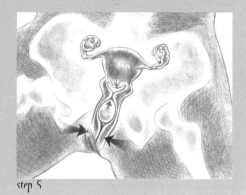

step 5

strengthening your erection

The strength of your erection can be influenced by the stimulation you are receiving/ producing for yourself (see pages 53–5), the strength of your pelvic muscles (see pages 72–3), what's going on in your mind, your health and lifestyle, and certain special techniques. The mental tricks that can help a man enjoy a better erection are described below. It's best to practise them alone because actual sex could put you off and lead to failure. These special techniques can also be practised as you masturbate.

● **Fantasy** Imagine a sexual situation in which your penis is huge and where your partner, or another woman, is delighted by it. Use whatever fantasy produces the biggest erection. For some heterosexual men this can involve another man. Don't let your internal policeman get in the way. As you stimulate your penis, lose yourself in warm, uncritical pleasure.

● **Visualization** See pages 66–7. Once you've created a non-threatening scene in your mind's eye, building up every detail of the place, do whatever you need to create a situation in which your penis is large and growing ever larger. Breathe deeply and enjoy the sensations of your huge organ. Once successful, you could go on to visualize an erotic situation.

● **Memory** Cast your mind back to a time in real life when your erection was really strong. Re-create the situation in your mind, enhancing it for best results.

your health and lifestyle

There are many scientifically proven ways to increase the power of your erection. Most raise natural testosterone levels in the blood, vital for erections.

● **Eat meat.** Lean chicken and shellfish supply zinc, needed to make testosterone.

● **Avoid milk shakes.** Research has found that men who drink milk shakes have lower testosterone levels!

● **Massage your testicles.** This will increase testosterone production the natural way (see pages 138–9).

● **Keep competitive.** Studies show that 'winners' have higher testosterone levels.

● **Exercise.** Men who exercise three times a week have increased testosterone levels.

● **Check medications.** Consult your doctor if you are on anti-depressants or drugs for high-blood pressure. Many other medications are also proven to impair erection.

● **Take time.** It's important to give yourself lots of time when training your erection. Try the stop–start technique explained in detail on page 62.

special techniques

Many men never achieve their best possible erection because they become trapped in less than effective masturbation methods. See pages 53–5 for lots of new ideas. In addition, the following are helpful.

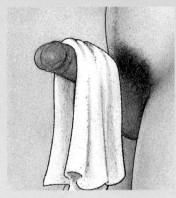

● **Penis weight-lifting** Men always laugh when I suggest this. But it works. It's basically a variation of the pelvic-muscle strengthening exercises I outlined on pages 72–3. Get a large erection, hang a small, dry face flannel on it (see left) and use your pelvic muscles to make your penis tip bob up and down. Then remove the cloth and adorn your organ with something a little heavier, or simply wet the cloth. It will be a lot harder to bob the tip. Keep going, re-invigorating your erection if it starts to flag. Add more and more weight over several weeks until your penis can stay big and you can flick it with some force with the weights removed.

● **Penis rings** These can help a man learn to have a hard erection, but they don't work miracles. Everything else needs to be working in your favour too. At the simplest level, you can improvise the effect. Make a constricting ring, using the forefinger and thumb of your free hand, and squeeze this firmly around the base of your penis (see right). Commercial rings must be used with care. They should be purpose-made for the penis (no curtain rings, please), you must be able to release them quickly, and never leave them in place if you have a tendency to fall asleep after a session.

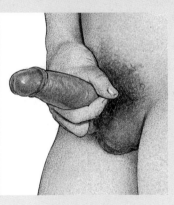

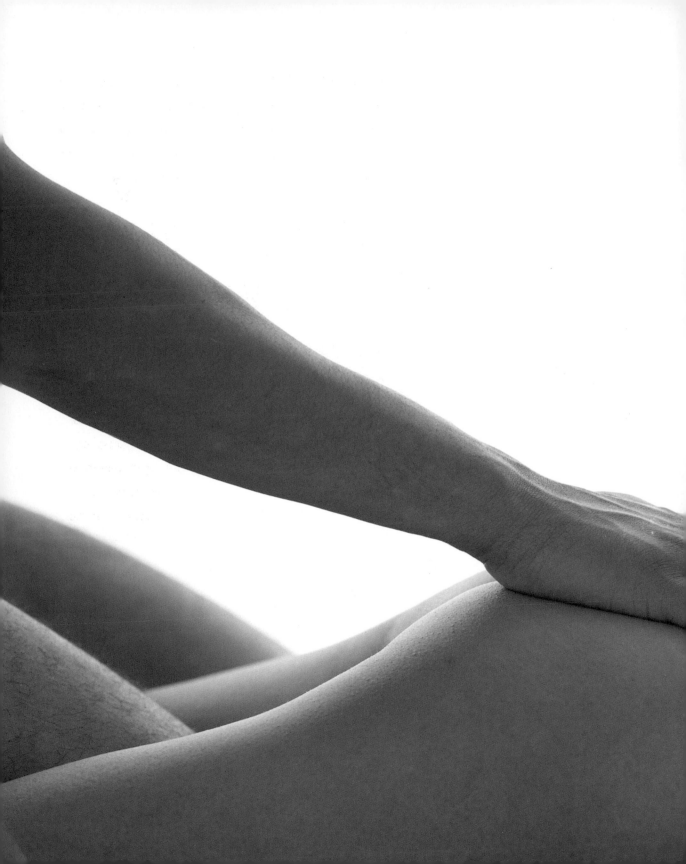

In Part Two I looked at ways you can enhance your sexual skills to strengthen the bridge between your experience of your lover and your experience of yourself. This self-knowledge is vital if we are to separate what we as individuals need to take responsibility for and what we can leave to our partner in any loving situation.

part three giving and receiving pleasure

Part Three describes many of the massage techniques you can use for fun, relaxation and arousal. But before you begin to explore, take time to look at the opening pages — on using all your senses, warming up, and breathing — reminders that relaxation and harmony are vital if you are to make a spiritual connection with your partner. In the many delicious journeys that follow I hope you'll find something to delight, fascinate and arouse.

introduction

Many of you who have come this far will have read books about sensual massage and will, of course, have built up your own repertoire of great erotic techniques. People often ask how it is that I have so a huge collection of such information at my fingertips, so to speak. Many say they imagine that my wife and I have long, thrilling encounters, involving hundreds of different massage tricks and pleasures ... and that I live out the contents of a book like this in my everyday life.

Of course I don't. Like a professional in any field, my greatest source of knowledge is the lives of others. I wouldn't be so arrogant as to write a book about erotic techniques based on my limited experiences, restricted as they are by my personality, life history, tastes, sensations and partner. But no one would think much of an accountant who gave advice based only on his own financial experiences and dealings. Indeed, it would be fascinating to learn how effectively bank managers control their own financial affairs! They certainly can't have run every type of business or coped with every sort of domestic financial crisis. Yet they are more than capable of giving sound advice.

Knowing how to respond to advice can be difficult, of course. Learning is always a personal journey, but learning what's erotic for you is an immensely personal thing ... largely because sexual and erotic pleasures involve so much that's unconscious. Many of our greatest pleasures arise from events and experiences that have long been forgotten by our conscious minds. Yet they are, nonetheless, extremely real.

Unlocking these delights can occur by luck. Sometimes, with an existing partner or (less surprisingly) with a new partner, we can experience novel sensations, perhaps after years spent believing we knew what best aroused us. But most of us most of the time need to do some deliberate, possibly guided, 'work' if we want a positive result.

Getting good at anything worthwhile in life usually takes practice. And this is where many couples encounter difficulties. Practising skills and pleasures – yes, you can practise pleasure – takes time and deliberate intent. But lots of people I deal with claim sexual pleasure shouldn't be planned – to be valid it should be spontaneous. There are occasions when spontaneity is paramount, of course, but once you've been together for some time – and especially if there are other things in your lives competing for attention – waiting for spontaneous pleasure can mean a long wait.

Those very same people will happily practise their hobbies, perhaps year in and year out, openly acknowledging that repetition brings increased pleasure and reward. Yet when it comes to their sexual lives they aren't prepared to make the commitment. I often ask them why. Finding answers to such an apparently simple question is, in itself, a revealing and valuable journey. If you as a couple decide to go this route, then be careful and treat your lover with respect ... the ground could be littered with land-mines! Be sure to remain vigilant and sensitive. Use your empathic listening skills (see pages 20–1) and really try to learn what's going on.

you are unique

Unfortunately, a book such as this – with hundreds of different types of erotic stimulation and pleasure on offer, many of them presented as step-by-step techniques – can seem at first glance like something of a 'maintenance manual'. But in the bedroom of any real-life couple the guidance it gives will be tempered by their unique relationship, their loving history together, their previous sexual experiences, their expectations, how they feel at the time, and much more. There are, though, a few thoughts worth bearing in mind in any erotic massage session.

Focus on your partner. Although erotic massage is, by definition, a two-way pleasure, bear in mind that when you are 'giving', you must keep focused on your partner rather than yourself. Doing what they love is the goal, not what gives you most pleasure in the doing. As you both near orgasm, this rule will, of course, be broken!

Make it personal. What you've done with anyone else is irrelevant. Listen to your partner and do what's nicest for them in that particular situation. Remember, too, that things change over the years, even with a familiar partner.

Be creative. I've tried to avoid annoying repetition when it comes to describing the erotic delights you can add to any massage technique. But always accompany whatever you are doing with other pleasurable forms of stimulation. For example, when massaging with your hands, also use your mouth, breath, genitals or voice. When caressing your partner's genitals with one hand, be sure the other is employed somewhere else. And so on. Although I've collected together many of the most popular types of erotic massage, I am limited by space

… and anyway you'll add your own special pleasures. I like it when people approach me in public and recount, with some delight, how they've out-done what I've written. If this book works as it should, you'll definitely find the same.

Use any – and every – part of your body. Although in the interests of space I describe largely hands-on massage, you can use just about any part of your anatomy to massage your lover – your tongue, your breath, your hair, your breasts, your genitals, your feet, your whole body, and so on. You'll be amazed how many delicious sensations are there to be experienced.

Assume nothing. When I'm teaching men massage, they often make sweeping generalizations about 'what women like'. The old adage 'When I assume, it makes an ass out of u and me!' is particularly meaningful when it comes to erotic massage. Making assumptions restricts your growth as a couple.

Don't limit your pleasure. Most of us today have puny expectations. There's no place for this with loving, erotic massage. The only boundary is your imagination.

sense and sensuality

To make a massage session really rewarding and fun, it's helpful to tune all your senses in to one another before you start. Here are just a few ideas. You'll come up with many others of your own. The idea is to create situations in which all your senses and those of your partner can be heightened and engaged. Reducing an erotic-massage session to a hands-on encounter misses out on a whole realm of delight and sensuality.

● **Water** There's a primitive joy to be had from water. Bathing or showering together can be a relaxing and sensual start to a session.

● **Food and drink** Feed one another delicious tit-bits or share a relaxing drink. Try not to overdo the alcohol – more than a little will dampen your senses and your arousability. Avoid a large meal before a session. Rather, if you're massaging during the day, make a meal together afterwards a sensual and loving event.

● **Burn incense or joss sticks, or heat aromatic oil in a burner.** Exotic scent can ignite deep passions. Or try activating your most basic smell centres with a pair of used panties and one of his worn T-shirts. Primitive, maybe, but nice!

● **Sensual fabrics** Fur, silk, velvet and feathers are ideal. Waft them, one by one, over your lover to create a gentle breeze. Draw them across their skin lightly but not so lightly it tickles or annoys. Place your hand on the fabric and, with hardly any pressure at all, move it over their skin.

Experiment on different parts of their body, using varying speeds and pressure.

● **Hot and cold** Splash a little cold water on to your lover's face or body. Run a part-thawed ice cube over their skin in long, tantalizing motions. Pass a burning incense stick or candle close to your lover's body so they can feel the heat. Massage with a hot-water bottle or a bean bag heated in the microwave.

● **Whisper sweet nothings.** Everyone likes to be praised by their lover. Say things such as 'I love your breasts';

'Tell me what you'd really like me to do to turn you on'; 'I can't wait for your thick cock to stretch me wide open'. And so on. Some couples like to use this as a time to compliment one another on their personalities, their kindness, or whatever.

● **Use your breasts or genitals.** Draw these sensitive and erotic parts over each other's body, asking the other (with eyes shut) to guess which part it is. A woman can run the inner wetness of her vulva down his skin. He can draw his scrotum or penis over her in teasing ways.

● **Use your tongue and breath.** Lick some part of your lover's body and blow it dry. Tease with breathy motions which alternate between tiny, quick movements and long, whole-tongued, languorous ones. Massage your partner with your hot breath, varying speed and intensity.

● **Use your hair.** A woman with long hair can tease and arouse her man by drawing it across his skin.

● **Use your whole body.** Sexually attractant substances are present in sweat, the secretions from around a woman's nipples and many other areas. Let your naked body become a massage tool as you surf up and down your lover's body. You can also use your arms and hands flat on their body to create a large expanse of skin-to-skin contact.

warming up

I make no apologies for using the term 'warming up' as if I were going to describe an exercise session at the gym. To get the best out of your massage sessions you'll find it better to start slowly, rather than homing in on some particular area of the body. Warming up not only helps you become attuned to one another, it also allows you to take things slowly at first.

OK, you may have a very specific 'goal' in mind, especially as you work from the book on any new massage sequence, but I'm keen to avoid the notion that this is a manual to be followed slavishly, step by step. Warming up carefully will put you in a mood that leaves both of you completely open to your unique journey of discovery. So use a warm-up routine like this almost every time, adapting it to make it your own.

1 Connect with your partner. Try kind words, gazing into one another's eyes, synchronizing your breathing, caressing one another's face or hands, or lying close and cuddling. Some couples like to read poetry to one another, sing a song, or even dance for or with one another. You'll soon discover what excites and interests you both. The idea here is to tune out the rest of the world. Remember: erotic massage is about the journey, not the goal. Your aim is to enjoy sensations and emotions at a really deep level.

2 Decide who'll be the main giver and who the main receiver for this session. This way, neither of you will be disappointed or angry after what should be a beautiful time together. Once this decision is made, the receiver can relax rather than being concerned about having to reciprocate the pleasure later. Of course receivers may want to reciprocate, but that's up to them. When you are both ready, the receiver lies face down, naked, on the bed or floor.

3 With a very quiet mind, lay your hands on the receiver's back. Then begin to move them, covering the whole of the back of their body with big, firm, loving strokes. This isn't any sort of formal massage – just a way of continuing to connect.

4 Keeping at least one hand in contact all the time, alter the quality of the strokes from deep pressure to gentle stroking.

5 Once you sense the receiver is relaxed, ask them to turn over and repeat the firm and gentle strokes on the front of their body, avoiding any obviously erotic areas such as breasts and genitals. If you like, you can 'accidentally' tease the odd glancing stroke against a breast, nipple, or groin but keep this to a minimum. By now the receiver will usually be relaxed and may even be starting to feel a little aroused. If you're both in the mood to take things further, you'll probably be feeling loving, connected and ready to turn to your objective for the session.

As always, it's vital to listen to any feedback. Be sensitive to the possibility that this is all that might happen in some sessions. Just because one of you wanted an erotic marathon, you don't have to go through with it. Freedom to change your mind is very important in such encounters. The loving couple who do lots of this sort of pleasuring don't get annoyed or disappointed if what promised to be a great session turns out to be a damp squib.

If it's you who decides that you want to stop at this point, take responsibility for the fact that you've started to arouse your partner, and do something to relieve their sexual tension. You could be lovingly supportive while your lover masturbates or you could stimulate them to a climax … whatever suits you both best. Remember to keep calm and friendly – no moods! There'll always be another day.

breathing and massage

Whether you are giving or receiving a massage, try to be aware of your breathing. We saw on pages 24–5 how deep breathing can help us relax, so, if you become tense or distracted, this is the way to bring yourself back to a focused state. The first sequence talks you through a technique you can perfect on your own, and the exercise on the opposite page helps extend this to create a profound connection with your partner.

breathing to relax

1 Shut your eyes. This will make it easier for you to focus completely on your breathing. In everyday life it's an automatic function to which we usually give little or no thought.

2 Take a very deep, slow breath in. The aim is to fill your lungs completely from bottom to top. Most of us, most of the time, never fill them fully, breathing only very shallowly with just the bottoms of our lungs.

3 Hold the breath for a moment or two and then let it out slowly until your lungs are empty.

4 Repeat steps 2 and 3 as many times as you wish. As the cycle becomes more familiar, you'll find that once your lungs are completely empty, they automatically begin the in-breath. Because the cycle takes much longer than normal breathing does, you'll find your breathing rate will fall a lot.

5 If you start to get slightly light-headed, don't worry. You're not hyperventilating. If you were, you'd be feeling anxious and experiencing pins-and-needles in your fingers or toes. Some people find that once they've relaxed into this kind of breathing for some minutes they are overcome by strong emotions that seem to appear from nowhere. Tell your partner if this happens and ask them to be with you, hold you or just listen.

breathing to harmonize

Great lovemaking might be described as stimulation in harmony, and breathing together is an essential part of that process. This sequence suggests one way to make a spiritual connection with your partner before erotic massage. With practice, it is possible to become so aware of your lover's breath that it is as real and forceful as the thrusting of a penis.

1 Place yourselves in comfortable chest-to-chest positions so that each of you can turn your head and bring your ear close to your lover's nose. Now you should be able to feel one another's breath easily.

2 Concentrate on synchronizing your breathing with that of your lover. This can be difficult if one of you is very much larger than the other – your lung volumes will be different and one of you may become short of breath at first. But with practice it is possible to breathe together.

3 Think about breathing the same air and gaze into one another's eyes. The eyes are the windows of the soul so you are now connected through the soul's two main gateways – gaze and breath. Add touch and you'll experience a togetherness and oneness that's hard to beat.

mouth and tongue

Although most people like kissing and being kissed, few do much to capitalize on the erotic potential of the mouth and tongue unless they are actually kissing. This is a pity because oral pleasuring is so basic, dating, as it does, from the very earliest days of babyhood, or even before.

Scans show babies sucking their thumbs in the womb, and it's a normal reflex to put objects into our mouths in infancy. That such experiences are in some part erotic can't be denied. Many mothers say their baby boys have an erection while being fed. Of course girls get excited too but the evidence is less obvious. And it's not just feeding at the breast (or more rarely, bottle) that babies find a turn-on.

Oral sex and kissing are the obvious adult manifestations of this ability to obtain deep, satisfying, sexual pleasure from our mouths but few people ever think of massaging the mouth and tongue as part of erotic play. They'll happily put their genitals in one another's mouths but not their fingers! Indeed, clinical experience tells me that many sexually together people have difficulty with mouth and tongue massage.

Of course, it can be completely unfamiliar, which is fair enough, but more often it has older, more primitive associations. For some people it is so intimate that they find it unbearable. For them it may bring back ancient memories, until now forgotten, of unhappy experiences when being fed – or perhaps not being fed – as a baby.

1 Once your partner is a little aroused (see opposite), ask them to lick or suck your finger. This usually causes few problems.

2 As they get more aroused, insert your finger further and then run it gently round the inside of their mouth and gums, avoiding their tongue. Ask which areas feel nice. There may be none at this stage, if things are unfamiliar.

3 Very gently run your finger over the edges of their tongue, and then play with the little band of tissue underneath it.

4 As arousal increases – you'll be doing other exciting things with your 'free' hand, of course – ask your partner to suck your finger while pressing it up against the roof of their mouth. At first this can feel tickly but the irritation soon subsides. Experiment with various finger positions until every sensation is pleasurable. Mouth and tongue massage is rather like foot massage. Done badly, it can be extremely annoying. But done well, it can be magic.

5 Arouse your partner more and more in any way they like, as you increase the oral stimulation, encouraging them to suck firmly on your thumb or finger.

6 Try a sword fight between tongue and finger. Some find quite vigorous contact highly stimulating.

7 Keep your finger or thumb in their mouth as you continue caressing with your free hand to bring your partner to climax (or ask them to masturbate).

Sticking your finger into someone's mouth from cold isn't much fun for either of you. Unless, of course, you're a dentist! So arouse your lover with kissing first. It's more than usually important to prepare your hands carefully too, and especially to make sure you have no infections or cuts. The receiver should brush their teeth or use a mouthwash.

As explained opposite, it is important to go carefully when trying mouth massage, always keeping tuned for feedback. It's a time for empathic listening (see pages 20–1). You could be amazed at what you'll learn and how this sharing can move not only your relationship but also aspects of your love life forward.

This erotic play can be an end in itself or a great starting point for learning the joys of oral sex, especially for those women who find it difficult to obtain erotic delights from the mouth.

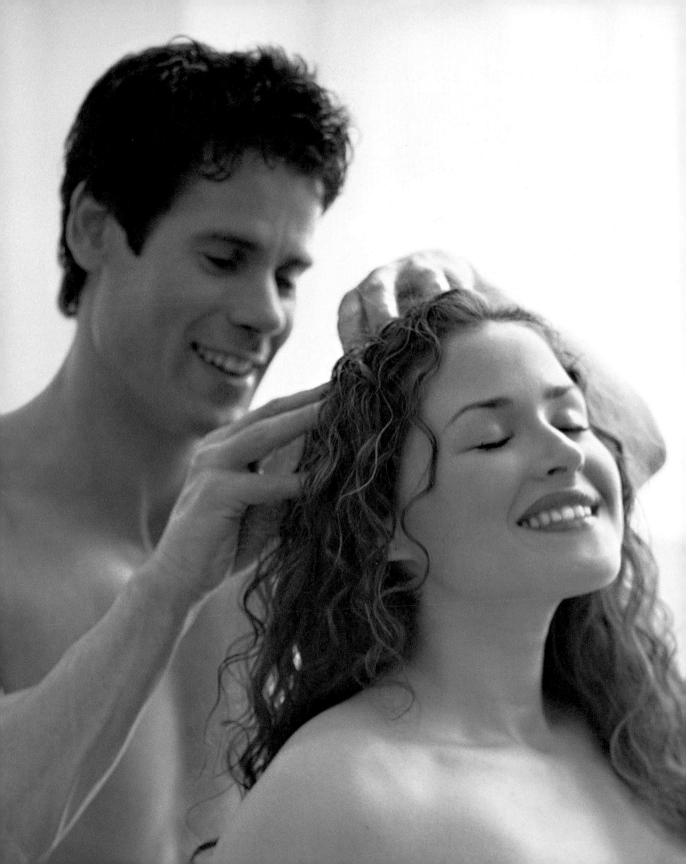

head, neck and upper back

I'm grouping these areas together because it's helpful to treat the whole zone as one. They are so close to each other anatomically that erotic massage for one can very naturally extend to doing something pleasant to another. And if you are the receiver, it can be difficult to be sure exactly which area you want massaged.

Many people hold a lot of stress in these areas. And tension in one can readily overlap to affect another. For example, tensions in the upper back and shoulder areas frequently go hand in hand with tension in the jaw. I'm especially interested in jaw tension because over thousands of hours doing bodywork with people I've observed that those who have tense jaws often have orgasm difficulties. Loosening up the whole neck and jaw area, combined with deep breathing that fills the lungs right to the top, makes a big difference to orgasms.

scalp

It is amazing just how soothing and erotic scalp massage can be if done sensitively. This is mainly because many of us tense our scalp muscles unwittingly. In the most extreme cases the tension actually produces headaches. But often the effect is more subliminal. Just use your hands for this sequence – few people like massage oil in their hair. Or how about combining the massage with washing your partner's hair? Lather makes it even more erotic. And you could shower together while you do it. Some people also find hair brushing highly erotic. You can try this alone or at the end of a scalp session, using a firm brush.

1 For a loving start, nuzzle your face in your partner's hair and run your fingers through it repeatedly as you stroke their scalp.

2 With each hand held to form a spider shape, use just your fingertips to massage their scalp firmly. Small, circular movements are usually nicest. Work especially over their temples and at the back of their head where it joins the neck – these are the areas most likely to contain tense muscles. Go very slowly and listen to where your partner says it feels best.

3 Vary the massage action by positioning your 'spider hand' in some of these places and just gently vibrating your fingers.

4 Make a small pad of two or three fingertips, seek out tense spots and gently massage them away.

face and ears

Although very few people have an orgasm simply as a result of having either their face or ears massaged, many say it's a great start on the journey to orgasm. But others feel awkward, or worse, about having their face and ears touched at all. If your partner seems resistant, take your time and be guided by what they like. It could take several sessions to feel at ease.

massage 1

It is best to have your partner lying face upwards, with you kneeling at their head, facing their feet. If you're not comfortable on your knees, you can place your legs sideways. Ensure your lover's hair is well off their face or it can be annoying.

1 Simply place your dry hands, one thumb to each side of their nose, palms down, so as to cover their whole face, including the eyes. This is very calming and helps even the tensest individual relax. Close your own eyes, focus on loving feelings for your partner, and slowly breathe in and out deeply.

2 Warm some oil between your palms (see page 43) and apply it to their face, avoiding their hair, eyes and nose.

3 Hold the sides of their face very gently as you use just the sides of your thumbs to lovingly follow the contours of the skin over their cheekbones, starting at the nose and working outwards. Work down to the jawline and repeat several times.

4 Holding the sides of their forehead, repeat this outward-stroking action as you work down to the eyebrows.

5 Repeat the whole-face covering action described in step 1.

massage 2

You could run this one on straight after massage 1, if you wish. Change position so you are kneeling over your partner's body – a knee on either side, facing their head. You can sit to one side if it's more comfortable. Take care not to exert any pressure.

1 Run a fingertip carefully and sensitively over their eyelids and eyebrows.

2 Trace the outline of their mouth with a fingertip – it will part slightly. Then gently stroke with the side of a forefinger outwards from each corner of their mouth towards the cheek. This can be a very beautiful sensation because it unconsciously recalls a sucking reflex from babyhood.

3 Plant masses of tiny kisses over their eyelids and ears, being careful not to tickle.

4 Gently suck and nibble their ear lobes. You may find this really turns your lover on.

5 Massage their lobes very gently, rolling and squeezing them between finger and thumb.

6 Run your lubricated finger around the outer edge of their ears. Again being careful not to tickle, trace around the inside of the ears themselves. This will probably feel unfamiliar to most people so go carefully.

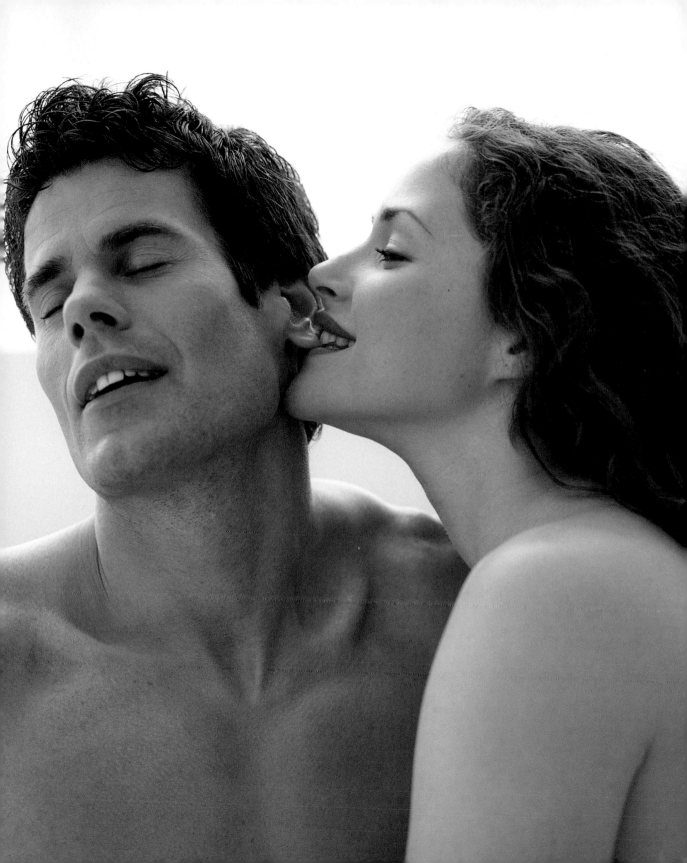

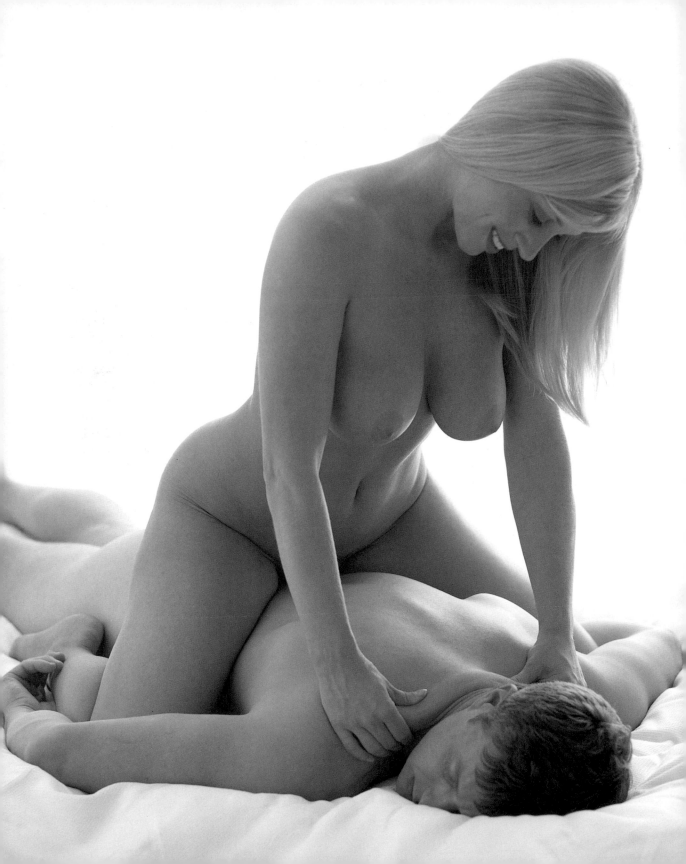

neck

Begin this massage in one of the positions used for massage 1 on page 92. From step 2 onwards, use the position described for massage 2 on the same page.

1 Starting from the mid point where the collarbones meet, slide your hands upwards simultaneously in a sweeping movement that ends at their jawline. Repeat this action all round their neck, taking care that your hands work together so the sensations remain symmetrical and evenly balanced.

2 Ask your partner to lie face down, and massage their neck firmly, using the tips of several fingerpads to make small, circular movements as you feel for tense muscles. Focus on any your partner tells you about.

3 Take the large muscles (see opposite) between the fingers and thumbs of both hands and squeeze or roll them as you seek out stress points.

4 Run your fingertips up the sides of their neck and into the hairline.

5 Plant kisses on your partner's throat, neck and chin, homing in on any areas they seem to enjoy.

upper back

For this one your partner begins by lying on their back. You might like to cover the lower part of their body with a sheet for steps 1 and 2 so they keep warm and feel comfortable. Sit or kneel at their head, facing their feet.

1 Place your hands, palms up under their shoulder muscles near the neck and gently knead the area. Many people find this highly erotic.

2 Again working under your partner's body, run your thumbs from the centre of their neck (avoiding direct contact with their spine) outwards towards their shoulder tips. This can be a very firm action. Although the position appears awkward, and the amount of movement you can make is limited, stay with it because your partner's weight helps you get good pressure here.

3 Ask your partner to turn over. Kneel at their waist, one leg on either side, facing towards their head, and simply place your hands on their upper back and shoulders. Breathe deeply, matching breathing rates as you focus loving feelings on them.

4 Cover your palms in warmed oil (see page 43) and massage the whole of the top of their back with big, circular hand movements. Go much slower than you think necessary, keep the movements broad and soothing, and wait for your partner to relax.

5 Working on one side of their body at a time, knead the big muscles that run horizontally from spine to shoulder between the fingers and thumbs of both hands simultaneously. Ask your partner to say what pressure is best. Most people do this type of massage too gently.

6 Run your fingertips firmly down the inner edge of their shoulder blades, seeking out any pleasure points. Many people say they feel aroused when stimulated here. One patient of mine talks of 'orgasms of the shoulder' when her man does this.

hips and thighs

Massaging the hips and thighs rarely produces an orgasm but it can stimulate exquisite sensations that are pre-orgasmic, especially for some women. The insides of a woman's thighs – from the backs of her knees to her groin – are linked by nerves to her genitals, and it is this that makes caresses here such an effective form of foreplay. For some individuals of either sex though, massage near the buttocks and bottom can be intimidating (see page 106).

For the sake of simplicity I've suggested the face-down massage for women, the face-up for men, but you can, of course, reverse them for yourselves. Cover the top of half your lover's body with a warm towel for these sessions.

When massaging the thighs, either back or front, always make the main pressure stroke upwards away from the knee, and the light, soft return stroke downwards. There are valves in the superficial veins of the legs that can be damaged if you force the blood downwards. It can also be uncomfortable if the veins are enlarged. Don't do this massage if they are varicose.

massage for her

1 Kneel between her parted legs, facing her head. Make sure you are comfortable.

2 Spread warmed oil (see page 43) over her thighs and hips, using broad, flat-handed strokes to cover her skin and make her feel loved.

3 Place one hand near each hip, just below her waist, and run them simultaneously and gently down the outsides of her thighs almost to the knee so that she experiences a balanced, symmetrical action. Remove your hands at her knee and repeat the downstroke several times. This movement is much more pleasurable downwards rather than upwards.

4 Repeat, placing both hands on one side and then the other.

5 Change position to kneel comfortably at her side, at right angles to her body (see opposite), and ask her to put her legs together.

6 Lean over her body and, starting at her waist with flat hands (fingers together) close to the surface on which she lies, draw one hand and then the other hand up on to her back. You are 'pulling' upwards on the skin and your hands should overlap to produce an unending wave of sensation as you travel down her side from waist to knee.

7 Switch to kneeling at her other side and repeat the procedure on her other flank. By now she should be feeling very relaxed and even aroused.

8 Kneel again between her legs but nearer her feet than before.

9 Run very oily hands up the insides and backs of her thighs, pressing quite firmly as your fingers form a flat 'platform' to flow up the backs while your thumbs massage the insides. Remove your hands at her bottom and repeat the movement, starting again just above her knees. Don't massage the backs of her thighs downwards.

10 Caress the insides of her thighs in any way she likes, teasing her up to her genitals but not touching them until you both decide you are ready.

massage for him

1 Do the wave massage described above (see steps 5 to 7), starting at his waist and ending near his knee. Make several journeys from waist to knee before changing sides.

2 Switch your position to kneel between his thighs. Using large, flat-handed strokes and plenty of oil, massage the insides of his thighs, getting teasingly close to his scrotum.

3 Ask him to bend one knee at a time outwards and massage his inner thigh. Run your fingers up near his bottom but don't touch his anus. You can massage his sitting bones in this position too.

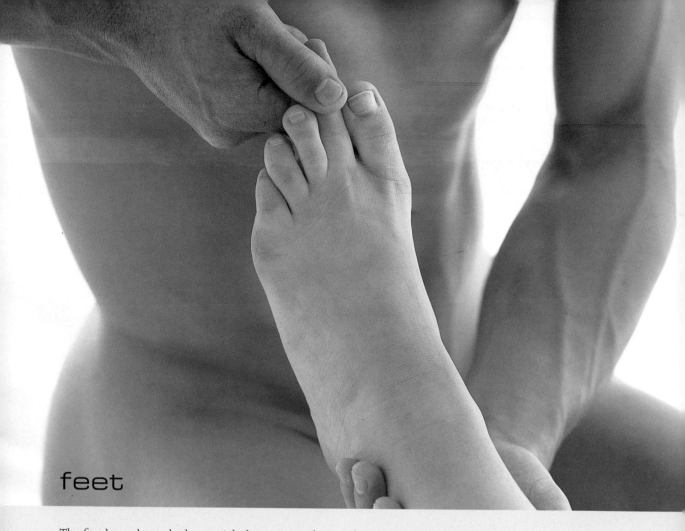

feet

The feet have always had a special place in sexual arousal. In Ancient China highborn infant girls had their feet bound because the folded-over foot resembled the female genitals and was considered very erotic.

For men and women today, foot massage can be pleasurable, even highly erotic. I have heard many women say that having their feet massaged makes them feel almost orgasmic, and some have reached orgasm from foot massage alone.

The main problem with massaging the feet, even for someone who finds it a turn-on, is ticklishness. Some people say that just the thought of having someone touch their feet makes them squirm. But this is usually overcome if the giver knows what to do. Indeed confidence is the key. When I run massage classes, people say the most annoying thing is someone 'playing about' with their feet.

If you are going to be the receiver, spend a little time beforehand making sure your feet will be nice for your partner to massage. They will, of course, be clean and the toenails short with no jagged edges, but pare off any hard skin on the soles too so they are soft and pliable. Nobody finds it very sexy massaging feet that are neglected. For this sequence, the receiver lies on their back, relaxed and comfortable, possibly fully dressed.

1 Warm some massage oil between the palms of your hands (see page 43) and then, using large, firm movements, cover one of your partner's feet with oil.

2 Hold their foot firmly between the palms of both your hands, placing one hand on top and the other beneath the foot. Close your eyes and concentrate on your lover's foot, channelling energy and love into it. Breathe deeply and slowly, matching your partner's breathing if you like, until you feel their foot and leg begin to relax.

3 Take their ankle in your left hand (if you are right-handed) so that you can support their whole foot in a position that's comfortable for you. Your partner must be able to relax in the trust that you won't at any time drop it.

4 With the thumb of your free hand facing upwards towards their toes, make firm, slow, circular movements, pressing deeply into the sole. Walk your thumb around, searching for places that your partner says feel great. If anywhere feels unpleasant or even painful, try elsewhere. You may be able to return here later.

5 Experiment: there may be other areas of their foot or ankle your partner finds arousing. It's hard to predict which spots anyone will find erotic, or even deeply relaxing. A favourite I've found, especially for women, is the inside of the instep. Run the edge of your thumb firmly with quite deep but varying pressure along this area repeatedly, using different speeds, until you discover what your partner enjoys most.

6 Push the fingertips of your free hand gently between their toes at the point they join the foot and then very, very slowly draw your fingers upwards to the toe tips, using the sides of your fingers to massage the sides of their toes. Repeat this movement several times.

7 Take one toe at a time between forefinger and thumb. Starting at its base, draw your hand away from your partner's foot as you gently pull on their toe. There's a delicate balance here between what feels alarming and what exquisite. Be sure to use plenty of lubrication, and listen and watch very carefully for feedback.

8 Finish by 'milking' their foot. Both hands are active for this action. Pull upwards on their forefoot, using the whole of first one hand and then the other, overlapping the movements so that you never let their foot go.

9 Repeat the whole sequence on the other foot if your partner wants you to.

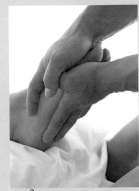
step 2

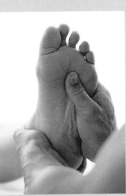
step 4

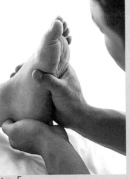
step 5

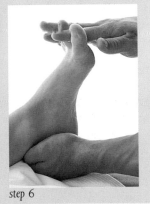
step 6

breasts

Breasts are highly erogenous zones for most people. Linked by nerve pathways via the brain to the genitals, they form together what I call the magic triangle. And it is this connection that explains why some men and women have their best orgasms only if their breasts are stimulated very actively.

Sadly many men, fearing it might be somewhat unmanly to admit to such pleasures, ignore or deny they enjoy having their breasts stimulated. Some even imagine that if they enjoy such games they might be gay. Of course, this isn't true. But for both these reasons many men find it hard to name the kind of stimulation they enjoy, so alien is it to them. A woman may have to be patient as she helps her partner relax enough to admit that anything feels good!

Naturally, as in every area of erotic massage, what each of us finds a turn-on or unpleasant varies a lot – even within any one person over time – but I find there's more disagreement about what feels good when it comes to breasts than there is with genital stimulation. The following observations should help when caressing your lover's breasts, though men will probably learn more from listening to their partners than from me.

● The breast consists of three parts. What feels good at the nipple might not be that great on the areola (the coloured part around the nipple) or on the breast itself. And what feels good to a woman at one part of her cycle may be positively annoying or painful at another. Keep experimenting and listening.

● Try not to make straight for your partner's breasts. Both sexes find stimulation in these areas much more sexy once they are aroused to some extent. (A woman's breasts swell considerably on arousal and men too notice their nipples enlarging.)

● Throw out any prejudices about what could feel good for you or your lover.

Many women are amazed at the excitement they experience when trying new forms of stimulation – some of which they at first imagine to be somewhat odd or even perverted.

● Most people enjoy gentle touch but some of the most overwhelming pleasures come from quite rough stimulation, particularly near orgasm. The nipple especially can take a lot of hard treatment without damage. But take care and be guided by common sense, especially if you are using clips, clamps or other similar devices.

● Just because something isn't instantly enjoyable, or hasn't been in the past, doesn't mean it never will be.

Because men's and women's breasts are so different I've divided the things you can do into massages for him and her. But of course there's a lot of overlap, and what one of you finds arousing the other may too.

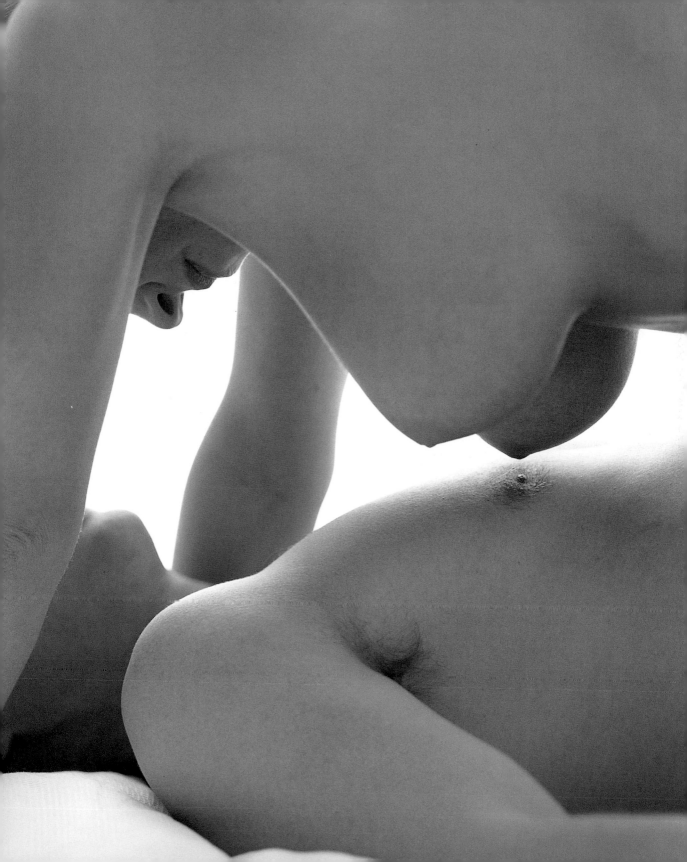

massage for him

● **Use your mouth.** Kiss his nipples. Take each one into your mouth and suck on it, gently at first and then quite hard. With the nipple still in your mouth, flick its tip with your tongue. Working first clockwise, and then anti-clockwise, massage each areola gently with your tongue as you stroke his chest or caress his genitals. Repeat, altering the pressure to a firm, deep probing into his areola. Gently bite each nipple and then massage it with your lips.

● **Use your breath.** Alternate hot and cold sensations by wetting his nipples with your tongue and then blowing on them gently. This can be delicious.

● **Use your body.** Lower your torso carefully over his chest and use your nipples to caress his teasingly. Then actually massage his breasts firmly with yours. You can do this simply by moving your body around, or by taking hold of one of your breasts and firmly massaging his nipples with yours. Try any of this naked and well oiled or through silk or some other arousing fabric.

● **Use your hands.** Massage his whole chest with the flats of both well-oiled hands, using large, circular strokes that reach right round to his sides. Gradually get closer and closer to his breasts and then, using small circular movements, massage around the nipple areas, avoiding the nipples themselves. Brush the back or palm of your hand over his breast or nipples repeatedly. (You could repeat this whole sequence with your feet if you like!) Roll each nipple between your finger and thumb. Flick it gently at first; then harder. Rub the tip with a fingertip. Take it between finger and thumb and squeeze quite hard until he asks you to stop. Pull out each nipple as far as possible and repeatedly apply pressure without letting go. Massage it firmly into his chest until it flattens or even turns inwards, against the bones underneath.

● **Use your imagination.** Find unusual ways to stroke or arouse his nipples, trying anything that comes to hand. Examples include fur, silk, rubber, leather, something rough, or a piece of wet ice drawn teasingly across them. Cover them with sticky food and lick it off.

● **Get rougher.** Squeeze his nipples much harder. Use a light plastic ruler to smack or flick the area. Bite them harder – being careful not to break the skin. Apply a clothes peg, domestic clamp or clip for a maximum of 10 minutes – less if the sensation is too great. If you are really keen, you could send off for mail-order toys or visit an adult shop for gadgets purpose-made for nipple fun.

massage for her

● **Use your mouth.** Almost anything you do to your partner's breast with your mouth and tongue will be welcomed. Start by licking and kissing various parts of her breasts, and then probe deeply with your tongue. Begin at a distance from her nipples, perhaps avoiding them for some time as a tease. Women say they enjoy this because it shows their partner has imagination. The underside of a woman's breasts is often ignored. It can also be fun to lie with her breasts hanging down above you: stimulation in this position will create entirely new sensations for you both.

Bite or gently nip the breast skin, covering her with mini love bites. Then kiss her nipples in any way that turns her on. Use the tip of your tongue to flick each nipple tip. Run your tongue round the areola, at first superficially and then very deeply. Many women enjoy probing here. Suck her nipples and massage every part of an imaginary clock face with your tongue, moving your head round as you do so. Press your tongue deep into her nipple, making it go inside her breast, and vibrate or pulse your tongue in this position. Take as large a volume of breast into your mouth as you can and suck on it.

Kissing and snuggling into your partner's breasts are also primitive pleasures that refresh old babyhood memories for many men. This is a delight heterosexual women miss out on, but the woman who is receiving such attentions usually enjoys it too, of course.

● **Use your breath.** See massage for him (opposite).

● **Use your hands.** Rest your hands gently on her breasts, hold them still and just feel your love pouring into them. Perhaps tell her something nice about her breasts, especially if she feels bad about them. Cover them with warmed oil (see page 43) or talcum powder and stroke them gently with large, flat hands. Don't forget to work right up into her armpits and around the undersides. Many women

tell me their partners focus too much on the central area. Some like breast massage to include the whole chest and even the armpits and the shoulders.

Ignoring her nipples, knead the breast tissue quite deeply, never taking

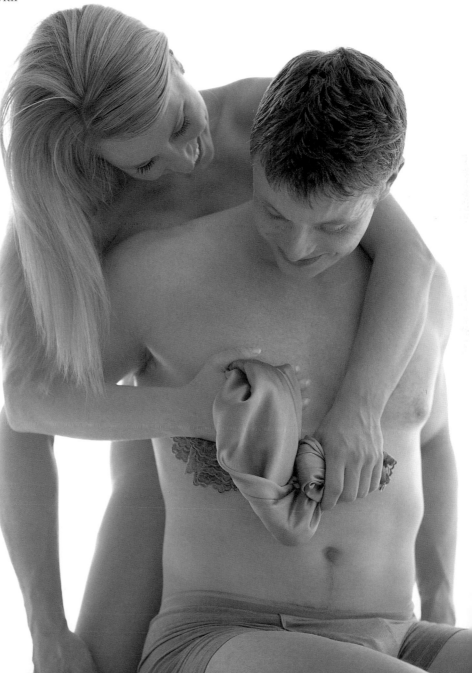

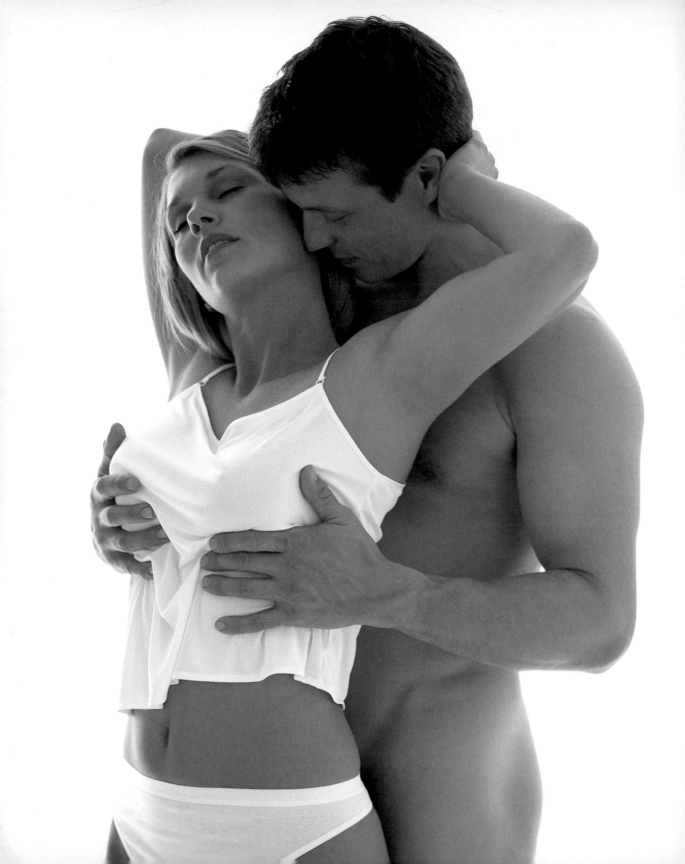

your fingers off her skin as you travel around her breasts – squeeze rather like shaking someone's hand; probe with your fingertips; and make small, circular movements with the pads of your fingers. Some women say they like their breasts being twisted or 'wrung'. Take a large volume of breast in one hand and squeeze it quite firmly. What you can do will be largely dictated by the volume and softness of your partner's breasts.

Experiment with various types of stroke and pressure as she guides you about what feels best. Be sure to listen carefully rather than going on your experience with past lovers.

Once at her nipples, try all kinds of caresses: stroke; flick; grasp firmly between finger and thumb and squeeze; grasp and slowly increase the pressure until she says to stop; grasp firmly and then pulse with more pressure, your fingers never leaving her nipple; do the same while vibrating your whole hand; repeatedly squeeze and let go; push into her breast and massage; pull slowly outwards until she says stop; pull out and twist – some women like this a lot. The possibilities are almost endless.

● **Use your imagination.** Almost anything can excite a woman's breasts and nipples. Silk, fur, rubber, leather are great for massaging her whole breast. Wet ice cubes are good too: drawn slowly towards her nipples, or placed in her bra at the nipples while you caress her elsewhere. Never forget that a woman's breasts are linked to her clitoris so stimulation there will increase her breast pleasures a lot. Cover her breasts or nipples with sticky food and lick it off slowly. Use sexy bras in your massage games. Massage her breasts through a favourite dress or other piece of clothing you both enjoy.

● **Use your body.** Oil your chest and massage her breasts with it. Using your penis, repeat anything she found arousing when you massaged her with your fingers (see below). Try this again as she hangs her breasts over your erection. Massage her with your feet. Experiment with any other part of your body just for fun and be prepared to be surprised.

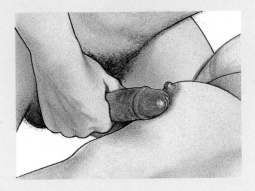

● **Get rougher.** While only a few women enjoy actual breast pain, many get very aroused by quite extreme nipple sensations. (See massage for him on page 102, keeping in mind the warning on page 100, and never do anything that breaks the skin.) You could also try hanging small weights from the nipples or applying heat or cold. After any extreme sensation, soothe her nipples with your lips, tongue or loving hands.

bottom and buttocks

What I mean by 'bottom' is the area that is neither buttocks nor anus. Massage here can be highly erotic for people who can't quite bring themselves to go the full anal journey. Because of this, it is very important not to 'accidentally' stray into or on to the anus while doing a bottom massage or you'll lose your lover's trust. I look at anal massage on pages 112–13.

If you or your lover feel somewhat unenthusiastic or even anxious about buttock and bottom massage, it is worth taking time to find out why. It's often a classic example of massage bringing up emotions from the past – emotions that need to be listened to empathically (see pages 20–1).

Many people are shy about showing this part of their body. They may feel ashamed because they have been brought up to think of the area as somehow dirty; they may have been smacked there as a child; they may have received childhood enemas at the hands of those who loved them: all reasons to colour attitudes to erotic massage in this area. But that doesn't necessarily mean they won't or couldn't enjoy it. So try not to run away from difficulties. You could do your relationship a lot of good by discovering what's going on.

Ask your partner to lie face down, ensuring that the top half of their body is covered with a warm towel. Their legs should be slightly apart but not so much that they feel exposed anally if this is an anxiety. If possible, sit at first between your lover's legs.

1 Warm some oil between the palms of your hands (see page 43) and place them on your partner's buttocks gently but firmly. Just hold them still for a while, breathing in time with your partner. Watch for the buttock muscles to relax. You'll also feel them doing so under your loving hands. Many people hold a lot of tension here.

2 Using both hands at once, work with flat hands in large, sweeping movements from the centre out towards the sides of their buttocks in increasingly wide circles. Press quite deeply as you go over their hip joints and linger there for a while, making small circles. This can create surprisingly exquisite sensations.

3 As your partner begins to relax, use both your hands simultaneously to make small, circular movements with the pads of three fingers at the point where their pelvic rim joins the small of their back. About 7.5–10cm (3–4in) away from the spine you'll find two delicious areas, one on either side. Stay here for some minutes. These energy points connect internally with the sex organs and can be highly stimulating.

4 Sit or kneel at the side of your partner. Take one

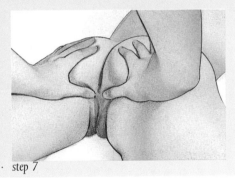
· step 7

buttock cheek between both your hands, the way you might a breast, and knead it deeply.

5 Sit between your lover's open legs and place your hands flat on their buttocks, your fingers facing their head and your thumbs on the inside of their cheeks about 5–7.5cm (2–3in) away from the anus. Hold still for a while, sharing your love and gaining trust.

6 Move your hands gently but firmly in a circle, pressing into your partner's bottom without removing your hands from the surface of their skin.

7 When your partner is completely relaxed about this, hold your hands still but massage deeply with your thumbs, feeling on either side for their sitting bones. Use circular movements, working all around this area and listening for feedback on which places are nicest. This could mean getting quite close to their anus or vagina.

8 If your partner remains relaxed and happy, you can go right to the edges of these openings without actually touching them. It's a huge tease and can be the start of a different journey, or an erotic end in itself.

perineum

The perineum lies between the root of the scrotum and the anus in a man and the vagina and anus in a woman. It is an interesting area because, although largely composed of the figure-of-eight muscles that encircle the openings here, it is also rich in blood vessels (see page 37) and highly sensitive nerves. As we become sexually aroused, these blood vessels enlarge, causing the area to swell.

Many people are shy or embarrassed about this part of their body because it's so close to the anus, something they associate with dirt and shame. Some men imagine that if they obtain pleasure from the area they might (or must) be gay, and are put off even trying. In truth, the perineum is simply an erotic zone that gives pleasure to men, whether or not they are gay.

Because of these disturbing anxieties the perineum is often overlooked or ignored by lovers. This is a pity because the erotic sensations it produces can be so rich and exciting for both sexes. Indeed, for the many women who complain, especially after several babies, that a penis in the vagina doesn't give them the kind of satisfaction they really want, perineal massage can be the answer.

It can also be a great halfway house between non-genital lovemaking and actual sex. Millions of women at any one time have just experienced some sort of genital-related trauma. Clinical investigation, medical 'manipulation', childbirth, gynaecological surgery, infection, rough intercourse, or even rape – any of these can put a woman off sex for a while.

But such adversities needn't spell disaster for her or her lover. I suggest after such events that a couple get back to non-penetrative lovemaking, with lots of kissing and cuddling, mutual masturbation and so on. And it's in this context of non-penetrative lovemaking that perineal massage can be so useful. Done lovingly, it enables a couple to prevent a temporary sexual setback from becoming a serious problem.

She should try on her own first, later involving her partner. If he is gentle and sensitive, she'll soon find she's relaxing as she used to, and her pelvic floor and perineum will be ready to take his penis, however large. Only when she feels completely at ease with her pelvic area once more should intercourse be attempted.

massage for him

For the receiver, this is a session to enjoy simply for what it is. It's best not to concentrate on obtaining or maintaining an erection. The only goal is pleasure. Lie face down somewhere comfortable and relax. Ideally the giver sits or lies alongside and leans across.

1 Massage his buttocks (see pages 106–7) quite vigorously to start the energies flowing.

2 Ask him to turn over. Stimulate his penis any way you both enjoy, just enough to get him slightly aroused.

3 With his legs wide apart, explore various strokes on his perineum. Begin with light pressure, listening to what he says feels nice. If this is all unfamiliar, he could find it hard to say what he does feel at first.

4 Hold his penis up with one hand and, starting at the base of his scrotum, massage down the length of his penis 'root' (see page 31) until you lose it. This may need quite deep pressure.

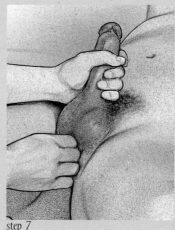
step 7

5 Press deeply, making small circles at the lowest point of the root using the pads of your middle fingers to stimulate his prostate gland (or g-spot, see page 114) from the outside.

6 Tap on his penis root or in his perineal area. Patting quite hard (or even gentle smacking) here is very arousing and can make a man come.

7 Make a fist of one hand and use your knuckles to massage him really deeply in his perineal area. But listen to the feedback, taking care not to hurt him.

massage for her

Make sure your lover is lying comfortably on her back. Her legs must be wide apart, possibly with her knees supported by pillows. The aim is to relax her pelvic and perineal area. A firm pillow under her hips will give you better access. Spend lots of time kissing and cuddling before you go anywhere near her vagina. Then caress her clitoris to ensure she's really aroused. She may be very wet by now but even so use plenty of lubrication before you begin the massage.

1 Insert the fore- and middle finger of one hand gently into her vagina. It is best to insert fingers in the vertical position (along an imaginary line between 12 o'clock and 6 o'clock). This stretches the perineum rather than the areas near her urethra or pubic bone, either of which can be painful if subjected to much pressure.

2 Gently turn your hand through a right angle so that your fingers are now horizontal, stretching her opening from 3 to 9 o'clock.

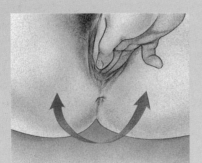

step 3

3 Press them backwards towards her anus and then sweep slowly and firmly back and forth along a U-shaped path from 3 o'clock to 9 o'clock. Keep up a regular rhythm, imagining you are 'smoothing out' the muscles around the back of her vagina. Concentrate on the outermost muscles. Your fingers don't need to be very far in. As this stretching can be quite stimulating, you may have to remind her to breathe deeply.

4 If she says that your caresses at one part of the 'clock face' feel particularly nice, zero in on that point, making a series of rhythmical, small U-shaped motions here.

5 Use your other hand to caress or stroke her in some exciting way and suggest she stimulates herself too, especially if she's getting turned on.

6 As she becomes more and more aroused, you can insert another finger and continue your caresses in the same way.

7 Insert all three fingers a little deeper (up to the second knuckle). Hold them still until she gets used to the stretch. She may feel like coming but don't let her – just stop moving both hands for a little. Take this opportunity to tell her how much it's turning you on. This isn't a gynaecological examination after all!

8 If she's eager for even more stretching, you can insert your fourth finger. Very few women who haven't had a baby can take this many fingers so go gently until you are sure she's happy with it.

9 When she's bursting for an orgasm, add your tongue to the game, playing with her clitoris as you keep up the rhythmic perineal pressure.

If you both enjoy anal massage, you might try these variations.

● Withdraw your fingers as your lover nears orgasm (step 7) – the tease will make her go wild – and re-insert three fingertips vaginally, the fourth finding her anus. Either stimulate just the outside as she comes, or push your fingertip gently inside.

● Ask your lover to kneel on all fours, her bottom facing you. Put on a latex glove and insert your thumb into her vagina, pressing upwards towards her perineal muscles. Gently hook the tissues outwards as you insert your forefinger into her anus. Grip the muscles in between firmly but gently, and then squeeze and roll them as you move your fingers in and out.

anus

The anus can produce highly erotic sensations when stimulated.
Unfortunately, many parents become over-involved in early bowel
training and we can end up feeling guilty or ashamed about our anal
area and even denying its pleasures (see page 108).

If you and your partner feel happy to explore this aspect of erotic
massage, some particular preparation is necessary. It's not reasonable to
expect your partner to indulge in anal games if the area isn't clean so
start by showering together, using plain soap and water
to clean the anus. Gently insert a soap-lubricated
fingertip and wash the inside. If you are planning
some sort of anal or rectal penetration later and
are concerned about coming into contact
with faeces, you can administer a small
enema. A pint of water is all that's needed.
Some couples make this routine a part of
their anal sex play. And remember: the
anus and rectum have delicate linings
compared with the vagina so make sure
your fingernails are short, or wear a latex
or nitrile glove.

When the anus is touched, it
automatically contracts, preventing
entry. This means that any form of
anal massage involves getting the
muscles to relax before insertion.
So give yourselves plenty of
time. My advice is to allow a
good half-hour for such a
session, especially early on.

Some people enjoy the sensation of the anal ring being stretched. If this is for you and your partner, there are two sex toys to explore.

● **Butt plugs** Start with a small one and use it only after you've inserted first one finger, and then two (see below). The 'working end' is tapered, allowing you to dilate the anus slowly and, once inside, the narrow neck above the other, flared end keeps it in position. Butt plugs can be used to stretch the anal ring as part of anal massage or as a prelude to anal sex.

● **Dildos** The jelly type is best. Insert only after you completed the whole sequence below. Your partner's anus must be very relaxed and open, and make sure they are highly aroused too, especially on the first occasion. With a dildo inside, the anal ring remains wide open. This is a novel experience and can be alarming so go slowly. Only when your partner is at ease, should you move the dildo in and out to massage their anal ring or rectum, or his g-spot. Combine these sensations with all kinds of other stimulation to bring your lover to orgasm.

1 Lubricate the area well with a water-based lubricant (see page 43) or saliva.

2 Use one fingertip to massage their anal ring with light, circular strokes, gently pushing on it without going inside. Most people find it helps to do this while caressing their partner in some other way. Simultaneous oral sex is another option.

3 Once their anus relaxes and opens up, it's time for penetration. Insert just the tip of a finger. You'll feel the ring tighten. Keep your finger still and wait for the ring to relax again. If your partner contracts and then relaxes their pelvic muscles, it will aid relaxation and help them get a better sense of what's happening.

4 When you sense your partner is comfortable, gently insert your finger a little more and again

wait for their ring to relax. Repeat several times until your finger is inserted about 5cm (2in).

5 With your finger still in position, help your partner to orgasm any way you both enjoy so they get used to the combination of sensations. This will also help to relax their anus still more.

6 In later sessions, concentrate on stretching your partner's ring, perhaps by moving your finger. In time you'll be able to insert more than one finger to make more interesting movements. (To find your man's g-spot, see pages 114–15.)

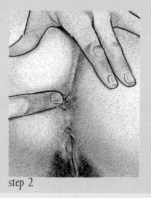
step 2

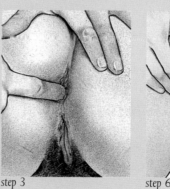
step 3

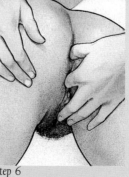
step 6

his g-spot

We saw on pages 32–3 what the prostate gland – the site of a man's g-spot – is and where it can be found. It can be stimulated from outside or inside.

However nice prostate play is, some men are anxious or guilty about any area related to their bottom being stimulated (see page 106). And many men believe women engage in such intimacies only to please them rather than because they themselves find it erotic. Part of the giver's job in a prostate massage session will be to help her partner relax in the knowledge that she isn't judging him.

external massage

Help your partner to relax before you start, perhaps by bathing or showering together. Then arouse him by kissing, cuddling, oral sex, or whatever turns him on. Bring him to several peaks but don't allow him to come ... keep teasing.

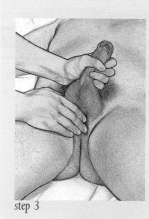

step 3

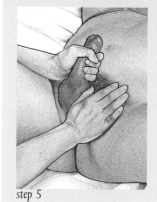

step 5

1 With your partner lying comfortably face down, his hips raised on a pillow or two, massage his buttocks and anal area (see pages 106–7 and 112–13).

2 Once he's nicely aroused and relaxed, ask him to turn over on to his back so you can caress his perineum (see page 109, steps 1–4).

3 Use your forefinger and middle finger to press deeply and regularly between the base of his penis and his anus once you find the magic point. He should breathe deeply, matching his rhythm to your action by inhaling and contracting his pelvic muscles when pressure is released and then exhaling 'through his pelvis' when you apply pressure. This will help him relax profoundly.

4 Make a fist and experiment with gentle knuckle pressure into his perineal area, listening to the feedback about what feels good. Try vibrating your fist. Or bring him close to orgasm and then use your knuckles to stop him coming.

5 Press the heel of one hand against the root of his penis, perhaps vibrating it. The direction of pressure should be upwards towards his shaft. Use your other hand to do something nice to the shaft.

internal massage

Some advance preparation is necessary if you plan to massage inside. It's wise to use a latex glove or a finger cot. You'll also need lots of lubrication because the anus, unlike the vagina, isn't self-lubricating. He can prepare by ensuring his anal area is clean. Some men use a small travel enema beforehand to wash out the lower rectum.

Many couples carry on from external massage to internal, if the man enjoys it. If you're starting with internal massage, be sure that your partner is highly aroused first and don't make a dash for his anus. Either way, take care and be guided by the tips on page 112 about anal massage.

1 Ask your partner to contract and relax his pelvic muscles as you put gentle pressure on his anal entrance.

2 Penetrate him with one finger. His sphincter muscle will tense so wait for it to relax. Wiggle your finger a little and then penetrate him further, moving upwards towards his belly, your finger crooked forward. You should now be able to feel his prostate as a firm, walnut-sized swelling at the base of his penis.

3 Press on his prostate or vibrate it with your fingertip. Don't worry if he loses his erection. The aim isn't to get or keep an erection; it's about prostate sensations. If this is his first experience, things may feel strange and even a little unpleasant.

4 Persist, perhaps over several sessions, experimenting with various strokes until you find what's best. Favourites are: a 'come-here' motion with the fingertip, applied with various pressures; a zigzag movement across

the prostate; and a vibrating hand action with the fingertip held still on the gland. Your partner may feel like thrusting his pelvis, quickening and deepening his breathing, or even vocalising.

5 Stimulate his penis with your other hand. As he feels he's about to come, stop caressing his penis and press firmly into his prostate. It might make him stop. If it does, repeat this cycle several times until he's begging to come. The more cycles of frustrated peaking you can take him through, the more massive his orgasm will eventually be.

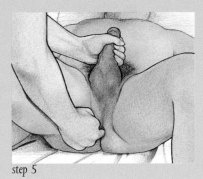
step 5

her outer genitals

Many men zoom straight for the clitoris or vagina once they start caressing a woman's genitals. This is a pity because they miss out on a whole pleasure system – her outer parts.

Before starting this massage, spend time kissing and cuddling and attuning to one another at a heart and soul level (see pages 14–15 and 87). Then help your partner find a comfortable position, lying flat with her knees wide apart supported by pillows and her bottom raised on another pillow. Kneel or lie between her open legs or at her side.

You will need lots of lubricant. There are many from which to choose. Vaseline and Abolene are OK but are rather thick and sticky and can stain the sheets. KY jelly is good but dries up over time. Keep a small water spray handy to refresh it. Various sex lubricants based on silicone are also available, and these are especially good for this massage.

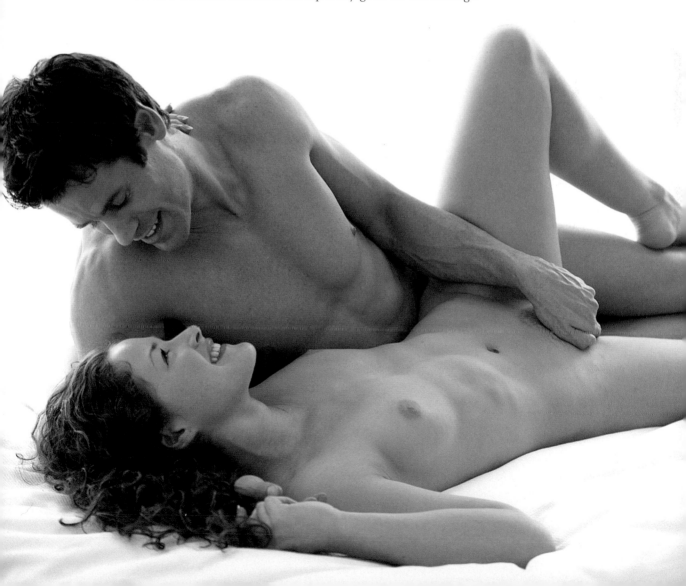

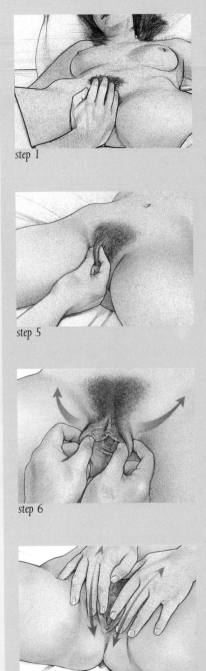

step 1

step 5

step 6

step 11

1 Rest the flat of your hand over your partner's vulval area, the 'heel' nestling on her perineum and your fingers on her pubic hair. Gaze into her eyes and synchronize your breathing.

2 With your hand in the same place, gently press and then rub her, making tiny circles, first clockwise, then anti-clockwise.

3 Move any stray pubic hairs before separating her inner lips by placing your palms over her outer lips and pulling them gently apart. In all that follows, avoid the clitoris.

4 Unless she's very wet, apply lots of lubricant. A nice way of doing this is to apply it to each large lip in turn, running the forefinger and middle finger of one hand up and down its length. Then use both hands together. Repeat several times.

5 Take one outer lip, and then the other, between your forefinger and thumb and squeeze and roll it firmly as you work from bottom to top. Then reverse your journey.

6 Starting near her vaginal opening, take her outer lips between the forefingers and thumbs of both hands, pull them firmly outwards and hold them there for a few moments. Repeat at various points along her lips right up to near her clitoris.

7 Hold her outer lips firmly and tug them alternately to an even rhythm. Then tug both at once several times.

8 Still grasping them firmly, pull quite hard to open her vagina wide. Hold it open and blow gently into it.

9 Repeat steps 7 and 8 many times, altering your grip along the whole length of her lips to create novel sensations for her.

10 Flick or smack her outer lips gently, being guided by what she likes.

11 Position yourself so your hands can now approach her pubic area from above. With her well-lubricated inner lips between the forefingers and middle fingers of both your hands, run your fingers up and down. This will pull deliciously on her clitoris (even though you're not touching it directly) and she might want to come.

12 Reposition yourself between her legs. Use one hand to part her lips so her vaginal opening is easily visible and caress the edge of it, paying special attention to the areas at about 4 o'clock and 8 o'clock (with her clitoris at 12 o'clock). Don't go inside at all. Just tease her and pleasure her in any way you can. Most women say they like firm pressure here.

You'll know you're getting this right if: her breathing deepens, she parts her thighs, she pushes down and out with her pelvis and arches her back, while her vagina opens up and seems to invite your fingers inside, and her clitoris (even though you aren't touching it) stiffens and becomes easier to see.

clitoris

Both sexes have a clitoris (see pages 31, 33–7 and 70), though most men are shocked to learn they have one. Many men with whom I've discussed this say they've spent a good deal of time trying to find their partner's over the years and to be told they have one too is amazing. If you want to get the best out of these sessions, don't rush into anything. Spend time kissing and cuddling before you start, and ensure you have good heart-to-heart contact (see pages 14 and 87).

massage for him

If your partner doesn't have an erection as you begin to massage, don't worry. In fact this sort of stimulation can be excellent for the older man who finds it hard to obtain an erection early in lovemaking. Erection or not, success depends on your man being able to yield to you as the leader in this situation. Some find this a lot easier than do others.

Help him get comfortable, lying on his back, his knees apart and supported on pillows. Then choose your own position. The main thing is to be comfortable so you can continue for some time without getting cramp. You could sit at right angles to him, sliding your legs under his so he can rest his knees on them and put the pillows under your thighs; or you may prefer to kneel at his side, with a cushion under your thighs, Japanese style.

1 Cover his penis with lots of lubricant or warmed oil (see page 43) and stroke it for a while in any way that pleases him.

2 Lay his penis flat on his belly and press with one or two fingertips over the little ridge where it joins the rim, massaging this area deeply until you find the right spot.

3 Try tapping it rapidly and repeatedly with a fingertip or two or vibrating it firmly with a single fingertip rooted to the spot.

4 Hold his penis head with one thumb and forefinger – your forefinger should be on the underside, over his clitoris – and roll it vigorously between them.

5 Place his penis rim between your two forefingers and rub them backwards and forwards simultaneously (rather like a boy scout starting a fire).

6 Lay his penis flat on his belly again and use a vibrator pressed deeply on to his clitoris. Be prepared for him to ejaculate without an erection, or just a partial one. You could stimulate yourself too by resting the vibrator on a breast or some other erogenous zone.

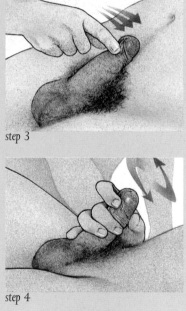

step 3

step 4

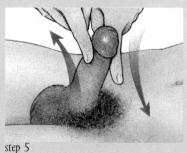

step 5

massage for her

There are basically two ways to stimulate
the female clitoris. The first is a long
stroke that travels along the side of the
shaft and then downwards a little further
on to the tip itself. The second is much
shorter and concentrates on the top half
of the clitoral shaft. Most women prefer
the second type once they are aroused.
Generally speaking, the longer the stroke
the more your partner will tend to lose
maximum excitement. Of course, this can
be a way of slowing her down or teasing
her, but make sure it's conscious intent
and not just sloppy technique.

    Right-handed women seem to find
most pleasure from stimulation on the
left side of the clitoral shaft. And the
reverse is true for left-handers. But be
guided by your partner on position,
speed, pressure and length of stroke.

    Dependability is the key to success.
You might get bored doing the same
thing for some time but it's exactly what
she wants, especially once she's really
excited. I've lost count of the women
who've complained that a man does just
the right thing and then 'fiddles about'
while she loses her high.

    Before beginning this massage,
arouse your partner in the ways she
enjoys, caressing her thighs, the backs
of her knees, her lower belly – anywhere
but her clitoris. And keep teasing.

    It might help your partner to get
the most out of her orgasm if she tells
you when she's close to climax. Many
women say that slowing down at the very
last moment helps intensify an orgasm.
Some find that as they near climax they
want no direct stimulation of the clitoris
at all. It's just too much. After an orgasm
your partner may want you to continue
so she can have another, or she might
want a rest without further stimulation.

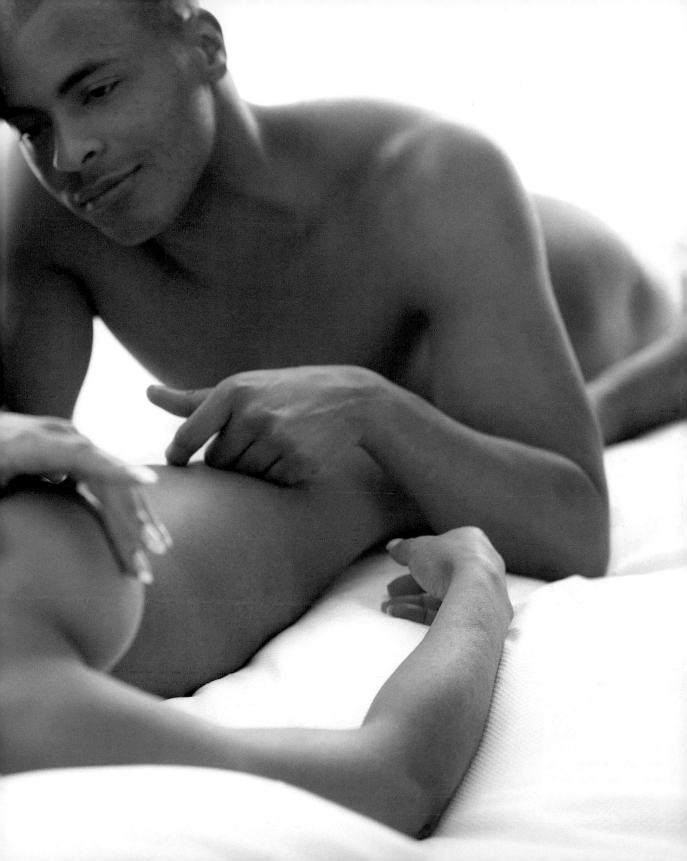

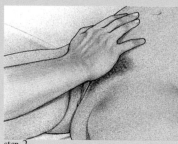

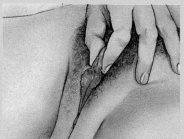

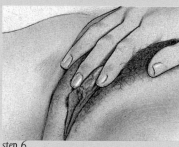

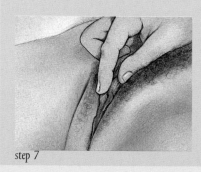

1 Apply lots of lubricant to the area but try to keep her clitoral hood dry so you can anchor it later without your thumb or finger slipping.

2 Place the heel of your hand (fingers pointing to her head) over her clitoral area and gently vibrate it.

3 With your hand in the same position, make circular motions, keeping your skin 'fixed' to hers while everything underneath moves against her pubic bone.

4 Pat or tap the area gently (avoiding the clitoris itself), varying the speed and intensity and seeing what she likes.

5 Using your thumb and forefinger, grip her clitoris at the point where the shaft disappears beneath the skin and roll it gently. It will feel like a very thin pencil.

6 Rub up and down both sides of her shaft at the same time, using a slow, rhythmic stroke and asking her to say when it feels good for speed. Many women say one stroke per second is about right. You can use a finger and thumb or two fingers for this.

7 Try rubbing up and down on one side of her shaft with your thumb while your forefinger makes light, circular movements on the other side. If that's too difficult to coordinate, rest your thumb motionless on one side as you caress the other side with your finger.

8 Hold the shaft between thumb and middle finger and gently stimulate the tip of her clitoris with your forefinger. Try this with her clitoral hood drawn back or through the hood for less intense stimulation. Many women can't tolerate any direct clitoral-head stimulation so sensitive are they there.

9 Grasp the shaft of her aroused clitoris between your finger and thumb and pulse (or squeeze) it rapidly.

10 Anchor her clitoral hood with your thumb and stroke her clitoral head with your forefinger, just as if you were picking up a very small piece of paper between your finger and thumb.

11 With the tip of your forefinger pointing towards your partner's head, use tiny circular movements to work your way around the 'clock face' very, very slowly, starting at 9 o'clock (with her clitoral hood at 12 o'clock). Discover what feels best for her and, when you find a magic spot, stay with it.

While doing all these delightful things with one hand, be sure that your other hand isn't idle. Women say several erotic inputs at once can heighten their pleasure and excitement, provided they are exactly what they want.

1 In the early stages, place your free hand beneath her bottom, putting two fingers on each cheek. This leaves your thumb free and pointing up towards her head: reposition it to lie against her perineum with its tip pressing firmly on to the opening of her vagina. It will give you good feedback on her pelvic-muscle contractions and you can use it to play with her there. Firm, circular movements are a favourite.

2 As she becomes more aroused, there'll come a point when her vagina seems to suck your thumb inside and she may be ready for you to insert fingers. You could try stimulating her g-spot or 'internal' clitoris (see pages 36–7 and 126–7) as you caress her 'external' clitoris with the other hand.

3 If she likes it, insert your little finger into her anus, or just caress the outside.

her g-spot

We have seen on pages 36–7 what the female clitoris is and on pages 122–5 some of the new ways in which recent research has encouraged us to think about a woman's arousal. Now let's look at the g-spot, a part of the clitoris that is easily stimulated. The g-spot is, in fact, one of several such 'spots' in the vagina. And they are all really parts of the 'interior' clitoris. Others are at about 3 o'clock and 9 o'clock, with the clitoris head or glans at 12 o'clock. All produce exquisite sensations when stimulated. Deep pressure can provoke delicious feelings that extend right down a woman's legs.

The name g-spot is, though, generally reserved for a very special area of the corrugated front wall of the vagina that 'appears' as a woman is aroused. Not only is it composed of blood vessels that swell on arousal, it also contains many small glands in clusters, like bunches of tiny grapes, that surround the urinary tube (urethra) as it runs in the roof of the vagina. As a woman gets aroused these glands produce a secretion that in some women spurts out as an ejaculation (see pages 128–9).

Many women like to start by finding their g-spot for themselves before involving a partner. Here's how. Empty your bladder and lubricate your fingers well. Naked from the waist down, squat on your haunches and insert a couple of fingers, palm up. Aim the fingertips upwards towards your navel and make a beckoning movement. Most women find this makes them feel like peeing. If it does, you've got the right place. If your fingers are too short, try a g-spot vibrator (see pages 68–9). Keep up the same action and see what happens … you know your bladder is empty so you won't urinate. The pleasure soon kicks in. Repeat the sequence lying on your back, perhaps after spending some time arousing yourself in the way you normally would.

finding it with your partner

Spend time kissing and cuddling and then, in whatever way you both enjoy, caress each other until you are very aroused.

1 Lie on your back with a pillow under your hips and ask your partner to insert two fingers, palm up, into your vagina (see page 110, step 1). Alternatively, you can lie on your belly with a pillow or two under your hips. Your partner now inserts his fingers palm down. Getting the right depth can be tricky at first, whichever way you choose. Let him know that he doesn't have to go very deep – about 5cm (2in) is usually plenty.

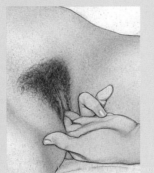
step 1: alternative positions

2 There are two ways to find the magic spot. You can ask him to start by finding your cervix (see pages 130–1) and then to stroke upwards with a beckoning action along the cervix and then along the vaginal 'roof' towards your pubic bone until he hits the spot. Or, with your clitoris head at 12 o'clock, he can work his way around the 'clock face' from 10 o'clock to 2 o'clock until he finds the place – preferably avoiding 12 o'clock because this could press directly on your urethra. Once there he should continue 'beckoning'.

3 Relax and leave the rest to him, though he'll need guidance on pressure, timing and length of stroke until he finds the combination that arouses you best. The sensations will increase if either of you presses firmly over your lower belly just above the hairline.

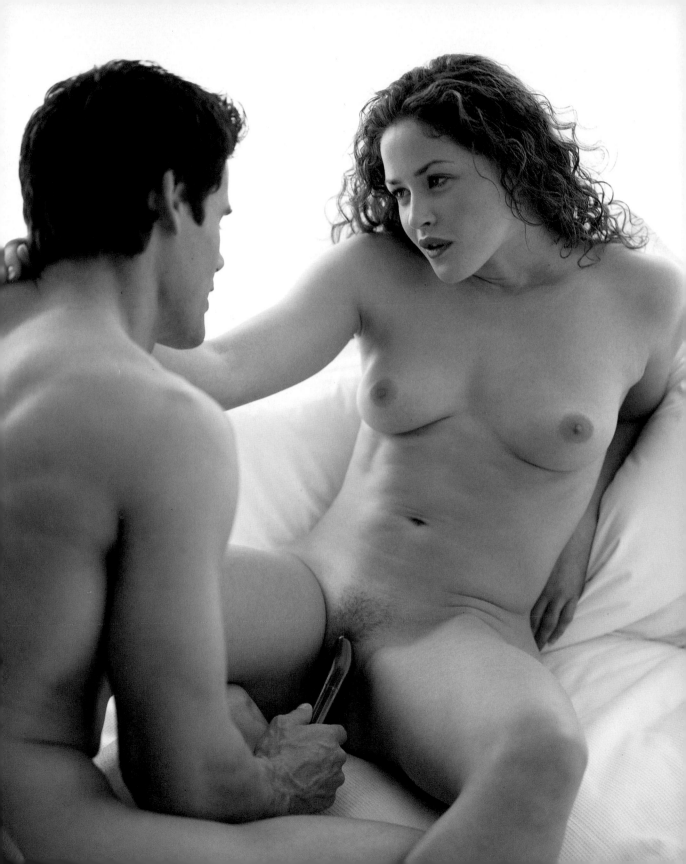

female ejaculation

Even today, there are few sexual issues that cause so much controversy as female ejaculation. Few people, including most doctors, believe it exists. Many women who are, in fact, ejaculating fear they are urinating, and either keep quiet about it or seek medical advice for what the average gynaecologist or urologist is quite happy to write off as incontinence. Understanding why women 'wet themselves' during sex, and seeking medical help, where necessary, can greatly comfort many women who are embarrassed by this problem. There are four basic reasons.

● **They are highly aroused.** Some women produce very large amounts of wetness, especially in the first half of their menstrual cycle. This perfectly normal phenomenon is welcome in most circumstances because it makes a woman's vagina more exciting for her and her man. One of the things many post-menopausal women and their lovers complain of is a dry vagina. A woman's wetness is the exact physiological equivalent of a man's erection. And we know how men celebrate their erections!

● **They are ejaculating.** When analysed, the fluid is found to be very similar to the secretions from a man's prostate gland. Many women's sexual lives are blighted by their ejaculation. They often fear ridicule or worse. But such women are sexual athletes, not sexual cripples. The days of men taking all the responsibility for the damp patch should be a thing of the past!

● **Their bladders are unstable.** Some women lose a small amount of urine as they climax due to poor muscle tone in the bladder. Peeing before sex can prevent this.

● **They lose urine in everyday life.** Such women wet themselves when they laugh, jump or cough, for example. Some find their bladders cannot hold on to urine for long. Both are forms of incontinence and need medical advice.

helping her to ejaculate

Ask your partner to empty her bladder so you'll both be sure any fluid lost isn't urine. Place a small towel under her hips to give her the confidence to relax and let go.

Once you've spent lots of time arousing her, concentrate on stimulating her front vaginal wall and g-spot (see pages 126–7). You can try using a g-spot vibrator, and there are also special g-spot stimulators that aren't vibrators. Most of them are S-shaped rods with or without a knob on one end. You may find she likes quite a lot of pressure. Take care if using any man-made device, though I'm amazed at how rough many women can be when they stimulate themselves to ejaculation.

She may want you to stimulate her clitoris at the same time, but don't find yourself between her legs caressing her orally as she nears orgasm because as she actually climaxes you could get showered. I've seen women ejaculate almost a metre! If she does ejaculate, be encouraging and tell her how excited it makes you.

pelvis

It's fair to say that most men don't get much erotic pleasure from receiving deep pelvic massage. The only area that's arousing for them is their prostate or g-spot (see pages 32–3), although some men enjoy anal, and even rectal, stimulation and stretching. Women tell a very different story. Some get pleasure from many areas within their pelvis. This is partly because there are quite a few accessible sexual organs in a woman's pelvis and partly because, when a woman is aroused or has an orgasm, almost every organ in her pelvis is involved. The drawing on page 37 shows the main structures of the female pelvis. For g-spot delights for both sexes, see pages 114–16 and 126–7. There are two other main erotic zones within the female pelvis.

Cervix The mouth of the womb or uterus is a hard, stubby, tubular structure that feels a bit like the tip of a nose with a dent in the end. Its size varies a lot, depending on how aroused a woman is. Nice things a partner can do include: stroking it firmly with one or two of their fingers; squeezing it between two fingertips; flicking the end; vibrating it with their fingers; pressing a finger firmly on the indentation as you become aroused; and inserting a fingertip into the dent (especially as you climax).

Womb This can be more difficult to find but it is moved when a woman's cervix (to which it is attached) is stimulated. If your partner presses his free hand firmly over your lower belly just above the hairline and tries to get his inner hand to meet the outer one, he can move your womb about. He could also try playing 'ping-pong' with it, batting it gently between sets of fingers.

Getting to the deepest parts of a woman's pelvis may not be that easy. Your partner will need long fingers and you may have to 'shorten' your vagina by squatting, or lying with your legs drawn right back on to your chest, your hips raised on a pillow or two. (In this second position, some women grasp their legs behind the knees and pull back.) Real sexual hobbyists may like to try lying face up with one knee either side of their head, their toes touching the bed above their head, and their back arched. In this position the vagina is fully open and facing the ceiling, and your abdominal organs fall away up towards your chest. You have to be pretty supple to achieve it but the pelvis is now open in a way no other position affords. This means, of course, that your partner must take special care.

Keep experimenting with position. You may discover one that, with the right stimulation from him, gives you huge pleasure. Working all this out can be fun. Everyone has heard of the g-spot but there are many other 'spots' worth discovering. If you ever experience pain (as opposed to unfamiliar sensations), ask him to stop. His explorations should be gentle yet firm and it's vital that he listens to you all the time, especially in the early days.

Before this type of massage, make sure your bladder and rectum are empty. Some women take a small enema beforehand, as neither they nor their partners like to feel stools in the rectum. A few couples make this enema a part of foreplay.

As always, it's essential to be sure you are highly aroused before your partner starts on this sort of journey and that he uses lots of lubrication (see page 43), even if you are aroused. Whatever he's doing inside you, he should add other stimulation with his free hand and, of course, you can caress your clitoris, or do whatever excites you.

1 Placing a pillow beneath your hips, lie on your back. Draw your knees up towards your chest, and then open them as wide as is comfortable. Ask your man to insert one finger, palm up, into your vagina, using the method set out on page 110, step 1.

2 Once you feel comfortable with this, he can insert another one or even two more fingers so you feel excitingly stretched. A few women can take all four fingers inside them.

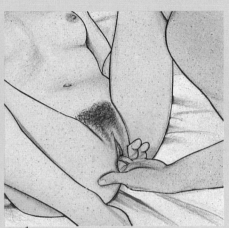

step 1

3 Alter your position, raising perhaps one leg at a time, so that his fingers can stimulate other parts of your pelvic cavity. Ask him to try wiggling, pulsing or even flicking his fingertips to produce the best sensations for you. In all these caresses he should be guided by your response so make sure that your feedback is clear. The sections on cervix and womb massage (see opposite) include other suggestions.

4 With his fingers still inside you, turn slowly on to your stomach, maintaining complete penetration the whole time. As you turn, you may discover other areas of sensation to enjoy. Ask your man to keep his hand still as you wriggle around to find the best positions for novel stimulation. Of course, he could use a vibrator or dildo to explore deeply too.

penis

Most men complain that their partners are too predictable when it comes to caressing their penis, claiming that the number of things they know, or are prepared to do, is far too limited. And, of course, this is often true. But, in a loving, open relationship, it is up to the man to guide his partner to an understanding of what he wants.

One of the best ways a woman can learn how to stimulate her partner is to watch as he arouses himself. Pages 52–5 also suggest many great methods of self-pleasuring for men, and one of the secrets of success is to know all the details. As any woman is aware from her own arousal techniques, it's the detail that matters.

Learning the skills of penis massage can be particularly rewarding for long-term lovers. Although a young man can, and will, get an erection with the slightest stimulation, most men over about forty find it more difficult. This means that a woman who has been in a relationship for many years may have to come up with creative ways to arouse her partner. Her reward will be that, once aroused, he'll last a lot longer for her than a younger man if penetrative sex is on the agenda. And even if it isn't, she'll love the hard, responsive organ that stays erect for ages.

But attitude is another very important element in great penis massage. The man should be relaxed, receptive and able to let go of the traditional male role as initiator of sexual pleasure. He needs to be able to surrender, to receive and to trust. Conversely, his partner should be able to relish her power and control in this situation, and to acknowledge that she's curious, aroused and interested in producing the very best results for her lover that she can.

It's a surprising paradox that some women of all ages can find this difficult. They may appear on the one hand very 'switched on' and sexually capable but yet still be reluctant to take control in this way. Most heterosexual women are certainly fascinated by the erect penis and the way it takes on its own 'character' when aroused but some tell me they find it hard to take responsibility for making things really great for their man. I suspect this springs from a deep, primitive belief that the erect penis exists for their pleasure rather than for their man's.

As with all the techniques described in Part Three, it's essential first to spend time kissing and cuddling, getting nicely relaxed and aroused. As the giver, take your time, and don't let your partner rush things. You need to set aside at least one hour for these sessions. Many men, especially the young, get so aroused as soon as their lover shows any real interest in their penis that they want to rush for orgasm, penetration or both. Teach him to wait ... but make the waiting worth his while.

Be very open with your man and tell him what you're looking forward to. Agree a word or signal he can use when he gets too close to ejaculation for comfort. You'll have to stop at once, perhaps doing the squeeze technique (see pages 62–3) to reduce his excitement, and let him settle without stimulation until he's ready to continue.

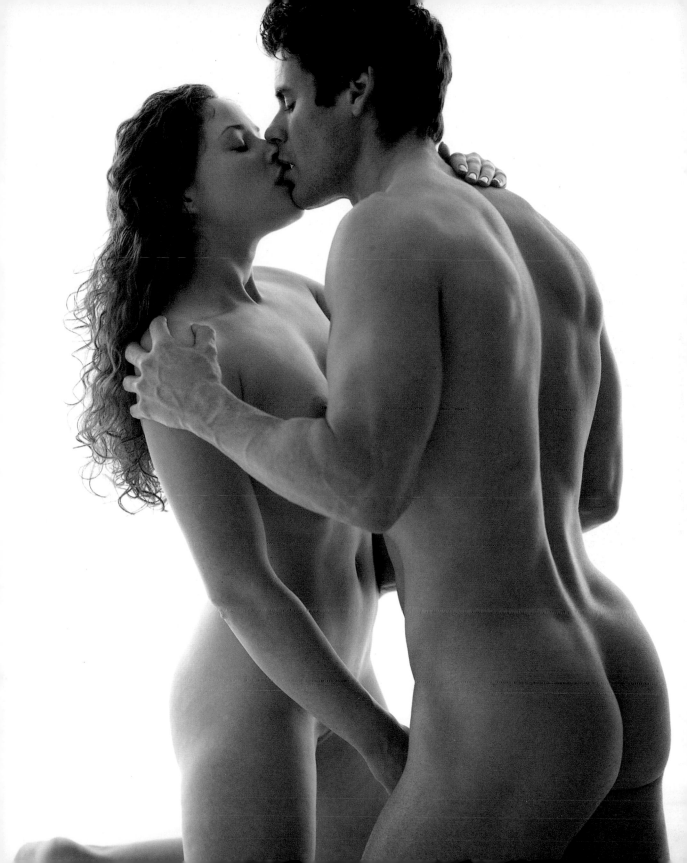

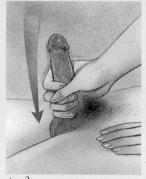

step 3

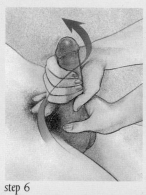

step 5

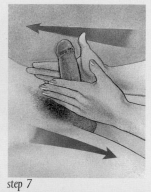

step 6

step 7

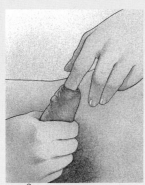

step 8

using your hands

You'll need plenty of lubricant from step 3 onwards. Water-based ones dry out too fast on the penis so use warmed olive, or a similar, oil (see page 43). If possible, prepare by helping him to shower, paying special attention to his penis, scrotum and anus. Then dress seductively: a man's arousal is greatly helped by visual cues. You looking sexy will be one of the best.

    Before actually starting the massage, have a long, sensual, chest-to-chest hug while you breathe deeply, matching your breathing patterns (see page 87) or connect using one of the harmonizing techniques (see pages 14–15). Then ask him to lie down or sit, resting against a firm surface, and find a position that you can hold for some time. You could sit at right angles to him, sliding your legs under his and placing pillows under your thighs so that his knees can rest comfortably on your thighs. If you prefer, you can simply sit or kneel at his side or kneel between his thighs.

1 Caress his whole body, encouraging him to breathe deeply with his mouth open as you breathe in time with him. If he has trouble relaxing, try some fun things, such as nibbling his ear or blowing on his nipples.

2 Cup his balls in one hand, touching his perineum with the tip of your middle finger as you press the heel of your hand hard against his penis root, over his balls. Place the flat of your other hand over his heart, gaze into his eyes and focus your love on him. He should open his love to you, filling himself with anticipation of what's to come. Together you are forming a circuit of love.

3 Move one hand slowly but firmly down his penis, pulling his foreskin (if he has one) downwards until it is fully stretched. Hold this down-thrust firmly for a few seconds, and then move your hand upwards, covering his penis head with his foreskin or your hand.

4 Repeat this action very slowly and lovingly several times. Be guided by what he likes best, modifying what you do as he asks for variations of speed and grip.

5 Lay his penis flat on his belly and caress it, stroking upwards, from scrotum to tip, using your palms and the flats of your fingers. Use one hand and then the other and lots of oil, working with a continuous motion so you are always in contact with his penis. Be sure to focus attention on his clitoris (see pages 120–1) as you stroke.

6 Secure the base of his penis with one hand and, with your other thumb and forefinger at the base of his scrotum, imagine you are unscrewing the shaft as this hand winds up to the tip. Use lots of oil on his penis head as you unscrew it. Repeat, with your thumb facing upwards.

7 With his penis between your palms, rub your hands backwards and forwards, working from the base to the top, and then down again. Repeat many times.

8 If he has a foreskin, gently pull it into place over the tip and massage through it. Then insert a finger under his foreskin and run it round and round the head, pressing into the fold where the skin attaches to the shaft.

using your vagina

Exciting though it is to massage a man's penis with your hands, he'll be even more delighted if you use your vagina. It'll probably be great fun for you too.

Although you can give your man a lot of pleasure if your muscles are fairly strong, the best results come when you can trap a pencil in your vagina while trying to pull it out. The first step may therefore be to build your pelvic muscles so they're strong and controllable (see pages 72–5).

To gauge just how fit your muscles are, it's a good idea to try contracting them on your own fingers before you do anything with your partner. Women who have trained to a high level are amazed at how strong the pressure is, and the experience teaches them to go carefully when playing with a man who is highly aroused. You won't damage his penis but it's wise to realise that too much pressure can cause pain.

Arouse yourself first, or get your man to arouse you, before you begin this session. You must be very wet. It makes a pleasant starter to ask him to put a finger or two inside you so you can give him a teasing taste of what's to come. Many men are shocked, and even alarmed, at the strength of their partners' pelvic muscles so this can also be an opportunity for reassurance. You'd be surprised how many men still think, however unconsciously, of the vagina as some many-toothed creature that could devour them. Such a man needs to feel comfortable before he entrusts his penis to you.

Once he's highly aroused and fully erect, it's time to choose your position. There are several good ones for this sort of massage. In any of the following your partner has the choice of staying still or moving too. Finding that combination of who moves, and by how much, as you work your muscle magic is half the fun.

● **You on top, facing towards or (see below right) away from him** A good one but make sure you're comfortable. Use your muscles but also move your whole pelvis up and down. Contract your muscles on the up stroke and relax them on the down; then reverse this. Try squatting over his penis too. This gives you almost surgical control over how and where to squeeze as he lies still.

● **On your side, legs drawn up to your chest, him behind** Nice and relaxing. Ask him to stay still while you contract your muscles and hold for as long as you can. Or contract rhythmically in an on-and-off motion. Try controlling the degree of penetration so you contract on his penis

head one moment and then further down his shaft the next. He'll be delighted.

● **On all fours, him behind** Only for the real enthusiast because it's much more difficult to squeeze his penis very hard when you are in this position.

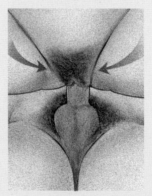

Using any of these positions and methods, play with his penis until he feels he's about to come. At a signal from him, squeeze really hard to stop him from ejaculating, taking care to listen to how much pressure he can stand before it gets painful. Repeat the cycle until he can't bear it any more.

You can also experiment with massage on his half-erect penis. Try inserting it into your vagina and then bringing it to a full erection by combining in and out movements with muscle contractions. A woman with great muscle control can do wonders for the man who fears that without a full erection a lovemaking session will be a dead loss. Of course, it does not need to be.

testicles and scrotum

A man's testicles and scrotum are easily accessible for erotic massage but what any man enjoys having done to them is fairly individual. Some like quite hard stimulation while many say a lover has to take things very gently. Certainly, if a man hasn't had an orgasm for some time, his testicles may be quite large, and you need to take special care because they could also be tender. The answer, as always, is to listen to your partner. He'll guide you to what he wants you to do, and you can adapt the suggestions below and build up a programme to suit you both. Oil (see page 43), warmed between the palms, is mentioned in only two instances but, in fact, can be used for most of these testicle and scrotum techniques. Or you can use talc, or nothing.

Before you begin the session, soak a flannel in very warm water to make a soothing hot wrap for his scrotum, adding 2–3 drops of essential oil to the water first if you like. Remove it before it gets cold.

● Gently cup his scrotum in one hand and do something nice to some other part of his body with your free hand.

● Wet the skin of his scrotum with saliva and blow on it. Then, if length allows, drag your hair seductively over it.

● Avoiding his scrotum, apply oil to the areas around it and to the tops of his thighs and massage firmly. If he gets an erection, ignore it, whatever he says.

● Work oil into his scrotum, perhaps using your nails to scratch the skin teasingly from time to time, especially on the underside.

● Push his testicles back into their little tunnels in his groin and hold them in place with one hand, while pulling down firmly on the loose, empty scrotal skin with the fingers and thumb of your other hand.·

● Roll one testicle, then the other, between the fingertips and thumb of one hand. Repeat several times and then roll both at the same time. Gently squeeze each one between your fingertips and thumb until it escapes (see below left), recapture and repeat several times.

● Squeeze different parts of each testicle, asking him to say exactly what feels nicest. Grasp that part firmly, constantly increasing the pressure as he becomes more aroused and giving one final, hard squeeze as he comes.

● Using one forefinger and thumb, grip the base of his scrotum to trap his testicles as a swollen, shiny globe at the top. Massage and perhaps tap (see below centre) or flick them.

● Lift his penis out of the way with one hand, using your other hand to smack his penis root. If this goes well, ask him to stand, lifting his penis out of the way, while you kneel in front or behind him and smack the underneath of his scrotum with the flat of your hand. This will give him exquisite and very different sensations according to where you are.

● Try a heat-producing skin rub as a massage cream on his scrotum, taking care to avoid his penis head because it would sting terribly.

● Grasp both testicles in one hand as you pull the scrotum firmly downwards (see below right). This one is most effective if your partner stands; you can kneel behind or in front of him. Go carefully so as not to cause damage – firm, continuous pulling is better than a series of jerking movements. He may want to masturbate at the same time, or you could bring him to orgasm with your other hand or perform oral sex on him.

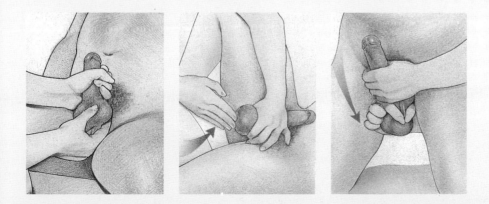

massage in pregnancy

Many cultures throughout the world use massage during pregnancy and birthing. This is almost certainly because massage acts not only on the body but on the mind. And during pregnancy many women find it helpful to balance body and mind as they prepare for their baby.

Couples often ask whether it's safe for the woman to have orgasms when she's pregnant. As far as is known, the answer is yes. It is said that very late on – in the last four weeks or so – an orgasm could start labour, but this would almost certainly happen only if the woman was ready to go into labour anyway.

Below are two special pregnancy massages for you to try together. You can use some of your familiar erotic massage techniques too: you could be surprised how different they feel now she's pregnant. But it's important to go carefully so use gentle strokes, be guided by what she says feels good, and read precautions on page 141.

● Your partner lies down for this one but if her belly is very large, she may have to sit. Start with your hands low down at her sides, pressing inwards gently against her waist muscles; release the pressure as you slide your hands upwards and inwards.

● Ask your partner to sit or kneel on the floor, leaning forward, her forehead on her folded arms, which rest upon a pillow on a bed or chair. It's important that she's comfortable so try it with her standing if she's not. She must relax her jaw and breathe deeply as you massage firmly at the base of her back, about 5–10cm (2–4in) from either side of her spine, using the pads of three fingers. Explore the areas with small, circular movements until she says it feels great. Some women feel orgasmic when this is done to them and many find it works like magic as a pain-reliever during labour.

preparing the perineum

Giving birth need not be painful. In the West we have come to expect that it will be but that's largely because we lie women down to labour rather than let them squat or walk around. When I was working with the Navajo Indians in North America I learned they had two words for 'labour'. One – for 'labour with pain' – was hardly ever used!

The better a woman prepares the muscle tissues of her perineum for the stretching she will experience during the final moments of birth, the less she will tear and the less likely she is to need an episiotomy. But it's not just these 'medical' advantages that convince me of the worth of perineal massage in pregnancy. Getting used to the sensation of extreme stretching is invaluable. A woman who has trained herself in this way can relax and actually enjoy the process. Many women say they wished they'd known about this massage before their first baby. Incidentally, there's little evidence that it's of much benefit in later pregnancies – but it's still fun to do.

The massage below is designed for a woman to do on herself. Start about six weeks before the birth, and do it for a few minutes at least four times a week. Clean hands and fairly short nails are essential, and, if you are worried that your nails may be rough, wear latex or nitrile gloves. Use a water-based commercial lubricant.

If you want to involve your partner in perineal massage, he can adapt the standard perineal 'massage for her' (see page 110) to suit you both. Most men very much like helping and many get turned on by it. It can, of course, lead on to lovemaking, whoever does it.

1 Sit or squat in a semi-birthing position with your legs apart. It's important to be really relaxed and comfortable. Many women perch in awkward positions and then wonder why they get poor results. Try to keep your jaw muscles totally relaxed throughout this sequence. I'm not sure why it is but a woman whose jaw is tight – especially if she is actually gritting her teeth – usually has very tight pelvic-floor and perineal muscles. Breathe in and out deeply and slowly, drawing air into the tops of your lungs on each breath (see page 86).

2 Lubricate your fingers and thumbs and the opening of your vagina. Rub the perineal area firmly for a few moments, working the lubricant well into the skin.

3 Insert your thumbs as deeply as you can into your vagina (up to the second knuckle, if possible) and use a U-shaped, sweeping motion with downwards pressure to move rhythmically from 3 o'clock to 9 o'clock and back again.

4 Roll and squeeze the perineal tissues themselves between your thumbs (still inside the vagina) and forefingers.

5 Hook your thumbs inside the vaginal canal and pull the tissues forward, just as your baby's head will do.

6 Apply steady pressure backwards towards the rectum. You will feel a tingling or stinging sensation. Keep your thumbs there as long as you can stand it and concentrate on relaxing your pelvic-floor muscles. Don't press forwards towards your urethra as this can cause irritation or even urinary infections.

precautions

● Apart from the lower-back massage opposite, any other areas of the body should be massaged only very gently during pregnancy. Keep away from swollen veins, don't do a whole-body massage if your partner has high blood pressure, **and don't massage her legs if she complains of pains in them.**

● Although some people suggest using essential oils, I'm not that happy about it. We don't really know how safe they are, especially late in pregnancy when the abdominal skin area is great and the absorption of the active ingredients so meaningful. Use plain oil unless advised by a qualified aromatherapist.

index

stockists

A wide variety of sex toys and massage accessories is now available from specialist shops, based locally or nationwide, and these can also often be a source of useful advice. For the less confident, mail order and the internet will be more attractive options. Indeed, for the most up-to-date information in a constantly changing marketplace, I recommend the latter.

My WHISPER vibrator (www.whispervibrator.com) has been designed to overcome all the criticisms women expressed in the study described on page 68. It is very powerful, yet completely silent; it is a pretty pink; and it has a smooth surface that is easily cleaned and self-lubricating. These features also make it the perfect massage vibrator for use on other parts of the body.

author's acknowledgements

I am indebted to my patients, who have taught me so much over the years.

publisher's acknowledgements

The publisher wishes to thank The White Company for the use of bed linen.